中醫藥文化教育（中英文對照）指導圖書
Cultural Education of Traditional Chinese Medicine
(in both Chinese and English) Guide Book

中醫典故

Compendium of Chinese Medical Wisdom

編　著◎許敬生
Chief Editor ◎ Xu Jingsheng

總主譯◎夏　昀
Chief Translator ◎ Xia Yun

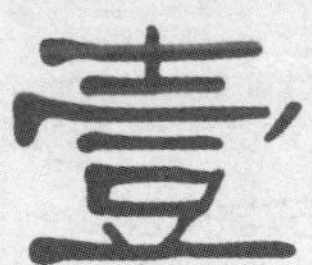

one

主　譯◎朱文曉　李　蕾
Main Translators ◎
Zhu Wenxiao　Li Lei

河南科學技術出版社
・鄭州・

图书在版编目（CIP）数据

中医典故．1：汉英对照 / 许敬生编著；夏昀译．—郑州：河南科学技术出版社，2015.8（2024.6 重印）

ISBN 978-7-5349-7703-9

Ⅰ．①中…　Ⅱ．①许…　②夏…　Ⅲ．①中医学－普及读物－汉、英　Ⅳ．① R22-49

中国版本图书馆 CIP 数据核字（2015）第 063917 号

出版發行：河南科學技術出版社
地　　址：鄭州市鄭東新區祥盛街 27 號　　郵編：450016
電　　話：（0371）65788613　65788628
網　　址：www.hnstp.cn
策劃編輯：馬艷茹　高　楊
責任編輯：李　林
責任校對：柯　姣
整体設計：張　偉
責任印製：朱　飛
印　　刷：三河市騰飛印務有限公司
經　　銷：全國新華書店
幅面尺寸：185mm × 260mm　　印張：14.75　　字數：300 千字
版　　次：2015 年 8 月第 1 版　　2024 年 6 月第 2 次印刷
定　　價：78.00 圓

編　著　　許敬生

Chief Editor　Xu Jingsheng

總主譯　　夏　昀

Chief Translator　Xia Yun

第壹分册　　主譯　朱文曉　李　蕾

First Volume　Main Translators　Zhu Wenxiao　Li Lei

名醫軼事 Anecdotes of Famous Doctors

情志之疾 Emotional Diseases

本草拾萃 Finely Selected Notes on Herbal Medicine

傳説故事 Legends and Stories

第貳分册　　主譯　孫俊芳　李曉婧

Second Volume　Main Translators　Sun Junfang　Li Xiaojing

醫史記聞 Records of Medical History

奇方異案 Unusual Cases and Unconventional Treatments

諷喻世情 Allegories Related to Medical Treatments

第叁分册　　主譯　穆海博　李　蘋

Third Volume　Main Translators　Mu Haibo　Li Ping

名句箴言 Illuminating Quotes and Maxims

大醫精誠 Doctors of Utmost Medical Excellence and Ethics

辨證論治 Differential Diagnosis and Treatment

養生健身 Guarding Life and Cultivating Health

第肆分册　　主譯　蘇　峰　劉　鴻

Fourth Volume　Main Translators　Su Feng　Liu Hong

醫鑒醫戒 Drawing Lessons from Past Medical Cases

雜説趣談 Miscellaneous Thoughts and Anecdotes

成語尋幽 Origins of Chinese Idioms Relevant to Medicine

破除迷信 Medical Explanations for Supernatural Beings and Phenomena

英文主審

English Edition Assistant Editors

Nicholas Phillips（美國）	Nicholas Phillips (America)
John Ruff（美國）	John Ruff (America)
Frank Phillips（美國）	Frank Phillips (America)
Evelyn Henry（美國）	Evelyn Henry (America)
王成至（中國）	Wang Chengzhi (China)
孫俊芳（中國）	Sun Junfang (China)

總策劃　　鄭玉玲

Producer　Zheng Yuling

總統籌　　鄭玉玲

Project Director　Zheng Yuling

策　劃　　張麗霞　徐江雁　許東升　徐恒振

Planner　Zhang Lixia　Xu Jiangyan　Xu Dongsheng　Xu Hengzhen

孫可興　張大偉　樊蔚虹　楊英豪

Sun Kexing　Zhang Dawei　Fan Weihong　Yang Yinghao

路　玫　尹　麗　郭先英　朱劍飛

Lu Mei　Yin Li　Guo Xianying　Zhu Jianfei

蘇　峰　朱文曉　穆海博

Su Feng　Zhu Wenxiao　Mu Haibo

統　籌　　楊英豪　尹　麗

Coordinator　Yang Yinghao　Yin Li

作者簡介

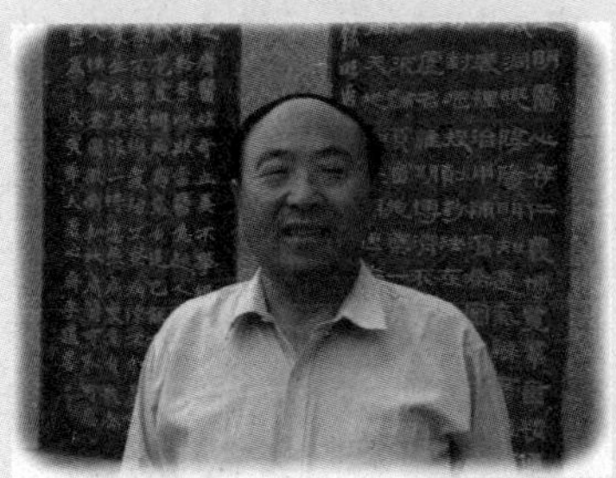

許敬生　安徽省蕭縣人，河南中醫學院教授，河南中醫學院中醫藥文獻研究所所長，中原中醫藥文化研究所所長，中華中醫藥學會醫古文研究會原主任（現爲名譽主任）、中華中醫藥學會中醫藥文化分會學術顧問、《中醫藥文化》雜志編委會副主任。

長期從事醫古文教學和中醫藥古代文獻及中醫藥文化的研究。先後發表學術論文70餘篇，主編出版了《醫古文選讀》、《醫古文語法知識》、全國高等中醫藥院校規劃教材《大學語文》、全國高等中醫藥院校研究生教育衛生部“十一五”規劃教材《古代漢語》等多部教材和教學參考書，主持整理了《危亦林醫學全書》《羅天益醫學全書》《中原歷代中醫藥名家文庫古代卷》等多部中醫古籍。

2011年7月，被中華中醫藥學會授予“醫古文資深名師”稱號。2014年5月，經中華中醫藥學會批准，被確定爲全國“中醫典籍與語言文化研究專家學術傳承與人才培養”首批專家。

Professor Xu Jingsheng is from Xiao County, Anhui Province, and is now teaching at Henan University of Traditional Chinese Medicine. He is the director of TCM Literature Research Institute of the University and TCM Culture Research Institute in Central China, Honorary Director of Chinese Medical Classics Council of China TCM Association, academic counselor of the Culture Council of China TCM Association, and deputy director of editorial board of the journal TCM Culture.

Having dedicated himself to teaching Chinese medical classics and research of TCM culture, Professor Xu has published more than seventy journal articles, in addition to edited volumes and monographs including *Selected Readings of Chinese Medical Classics* and *Grammar of Classical Chinese Medical Texts*. He is the editor-in-chief of *Classical Chinese*, a textbook project undertaken by the Ministry of Health. He also collected, edited and published ancient medical classics including *Wei Yilin's Medical Encyclopedia* , *Luo Tianyi's Medical Encyclopedia* and *Works of Central Chinese TCM Masters · Ancient Period Volume* .

In July, 2011, Prof. Xu received from China TCM Association the honorary title of “Senior Professor of Chinese Medical Classics.” He is also among the first group of scholars approved by the China TCM Association to participate in the “Chinese Medical Classics, Linguistics and Cultural Studies” research project.

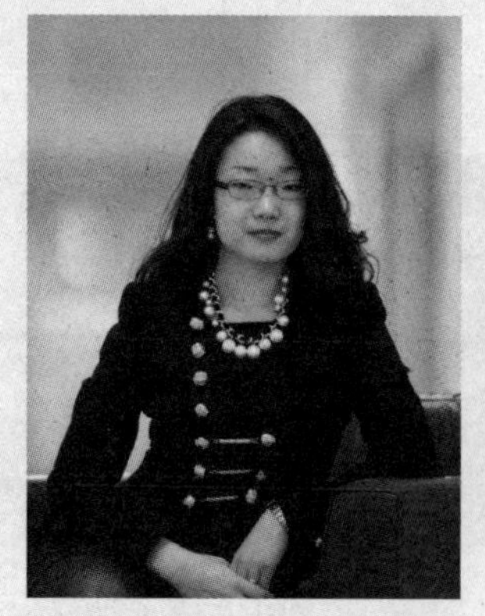

夏昀 2004年畢業於北京大學，獲歷史學與經濟學雙學士，並於當年到美國俄勒岡大學碩博連讀，2010年畢業獲博士學位。2010年8月至2012年8月任教于美國西雅圖大學，2012年9月至今任教于美國瓦爾帕萊索大學。主講東亞歷史、近現代史、亞洲電影欣賞、世界史、中日關係史等課程，並曾受邀至華盛頓大學、哥倫比亞大學等著名學府做學術報告。

夏昀博士在研究東亞法制史之餘，對東西方電影及其發展史頗感興趣，曾在美國其所任教的高等學府開設“電影裏的現代中國”及“東亞國家電影史”等課程。夏昀博士更致力于翻譯和推介反映中國傳統文化和歷史的優秀電影，由她擔任英文主譯的《蒼生大醫》《精誠大醫》《電影兒女》等多部電影已經在國內外公映。她主譯的大型歷史舞臺戲劇《蘇武牧羊》于2012年3月8日在北京人民大會堂上映，中國國家領導人和三十六個國家駐中國大使館的大使共同觀賞了該劇，各國大使對劇中優美的英文翻譯給與了高度贊揚。2012年，《蘇武牧羊》獲中國最高戲曲獎。

Dr. Xia Yun holds a Ph.D. degree from the University of Oregon (2010), having earned her B.A. degree in History and Economics from Beijing University (2004). She taught at Seattle University from 2010 to 2012, and since 2012 has been assistant professor of history at Valparaiso University, Indiana. She regularly offers courses on East Asian history and culture, film studies, world history, China-Japan relations, law and society in China, and other topics. She has been invited to give guest lectures and share her research at the University of Washington and Columbia University, among other institutions.

Dr. Xia's research focuses on Chinese legal history, although she is interested in a variety of academic and cultural subjects. She has a passion for film studies, and has taught film courses including "Modern China through Film" and "Organized Crime in Asia through Film". In addition, she has provided English subtitles for several Chinese films, including *People's Doctor* (2006), and *A Great Master of Chinese Medicine* (2011). She also translated the scripts of the historical play "*Su Wu: Story of a Chinese Diplomat*", which was on stage in March, 2012 at the Great Hall of the People and was well received among Chinese dignitaries and foreign ambassadors.

序言

中醫隨中華民族的誕生而誕生，伴中華民族的繁衍而發展。數千年積籍浩瀚，聖賢典故、凡醫趣聞、豐富多彩。而賞者衆，集者鮮。

許敬生老師，學本文史，授課醫古文數十年，成就斐然。年逾古稀，仍精勤不倦，博覽群書，廣勘闊采，展卷百數，選録典故、軼事。涉醫、文、史，輯爲《中醫典故》，列分醫史記聞，大醫精誠，養生健身，名醫軼事，名句箴言，醫鑒醫戒，辨證論治，奇方異案，雜説趣談等，凡十五類。書成，有幸先睹，覽勝喟嘆：豈止中醫典故？所涉廣博。豈止寓教醫者？更啓世人知醫。豈止學者興致？信雅俗共賞。豈止益享國人？異域亦必争覽。偶生一念：譯爲外文，共賞天下，焉非佳冀？

商諸老師，欣然同意。于是特邀美國瓦爾帕萊索大學歷史系助理教授夏昀博士爲主譯，邀美國伊利諾伊州大學法學博士 Nicholas Phillips，美國瓦爾帕萊索大學英語系教授 John Ruff 博士，美國布朗大學醫學博士、聖盧克醫院執業醫師 Evelyn Henry，美國聖瑪麗私立學校校長 Frank Phillips 先生，上海社會科學院王成至教授及河南中醫學院的孫俊芳教授爲主審，皆應邀協力，切意翻譯，英文版將付梓，是序也。

鄭玉玲

河南中醫學院院長

2014 年 7 月

Preface

The development of Chinese civilization has been accompanied and punctuated by the flourishing of Traditional Chinese Medicine. The indigenous medical theories and practices in China ensured the proliferation of the Chinese people. Over the past thousands of years, a vast amount of classic texts, anecdotes, pieces of ancient wisdom, and stories of renowned doctors piled up into a rich repository of knowledge. Many have read and appreciated such materials, and yet few collect and compile them.

Prof. Xu Jingsheng had taught classic Chinese medical texts for decades and is a leading authority in this field. With an outstanding education in liberal arts, Professor Xu continues to read and write diligently at an age of over seventy. He browsed through hundreds of volumes of medical, literary and historical works, searching for valuable pieces on philosophies and practices of TCM. What comes out of this ambitious project is *Compendium of Chinese Medical Wisdom*. This work contains fifteen categories including the follows: *Records of Medical History*, *Medical Ethics and Skills of Great Doctors*, *Health Cultivation and Body Building*, *Anecdotes of Renowned Doctors*, *Famous Maxims*, *Unusual Cases and Unconventional Treatments*, *Lessons and Warnings for Physicians*, *Syndrome Differentiation and Treatment*, and Miscellany. Upon its completion, I had the honor to be the first reader of the book. I was deeply impressed by how profound and comprehensive the content is. This book goes beyond a collection of excerpts and quotations about Chinese medicine, and takes readers into all different realms of Chinese culture. Not only is it beneficial to medical practitioners, it will also enlighten people from all walks of life regarding the world of medicine. This work is serious enough for scholars, yet accessible enough for a larger audience. It will prove intriguing for Chinese and foreigners alike. For such reasons, I suggested translating it into English and sharing it with a much larger community.

Prof. Xu was delighted to hear this suggestion. We thus invited Dr. Xia Yun, assistant professor of History at Valparaiso University to be the chief translator. Also on the translation team are: Dr. John Ruff, professor of English from Valparaiso University, Mr. Nicholas Phillips, a J.D. from University of Illinois, Dr. Evelyn Henry, a graduate of Brown University medical school who now practices at St. Luke's Hospital, Mr. Frank Phillips, the principal of Saint Mary's School in the USA, and Dr. Wang Chengzhi from Shanghai Academy of Social Sciences，Sun Junfang from Henan University of TCM. Now that the English version is going to be published soon, I hereby laud their joint efforts.

Zheng Yuling

President of Henan University of TCM

July 2014

前　言

在浩如煙海的古代醫學著作和其他古籍中，保存了許多有關醫家和中醫藥知識的典故。這些典故發人深思，啓迪智慧，且詼諧幽默，充滿了知識性和趣味性，頗有教育意義。對學習古代漢語及提高閱讀古醫籍的能力，也大有幫助。而有關這方面的知識，當今介紹甚少。多年來，我在閱讀古書的過程中，留心收集了不少資料，初步進行了這方面的研究，深感其中蘊蓄着精深的中醫藥文化和豐富的語言寶藏。於是奮編摩之志，决心在整理醫林中流傳已久的典故的基礎上，同時總結歸納古籍中有關醫學的若干典故資料，以便提煉出新的成語典故，供社會流傳使用，進而豐富祖國的語言寶庫。

成語典故是經過人們長期使用、反復加工錘煉而形成的結構相對固定的詞語或短語。往往具備語音和諧、結構整齊、語義含蓄、語言生動等特點，是語言中的精華。許多現代人正是通過對漢語中的成語典故的學習和使用，而在一定程度上保留了對逐漸生疏的古代漢語的一些記憶。

衆所周知，成語典故來源於古代的典籍、詩文雜記和民間的俚語、諺語等，而作爲與人的生命、生活休戚相關的中醫藥學，自然也是成語典故的源頭之一。本書也收載了一些流傳已久的與中醫藥有關的或直接來源於醫學著作的成語典故，如膏肓、吐故納新、對症下藥、樂極生悲、不可救藥、流水不腐、户樞不螻（蠹）、三折肱知爲良醫等。這些成語典故，不僅保留着醫藥學的意義，而且早已延伸到更廣泛的社會領域，用以説明一些社會現象，因而具備了廣泛的社會學意義。這類成語典故在應用的過程中，醫學和社會學相互滲透而廣泛聯繫的現象，充分體現了中醫藥學的發展和普及，也體現了社會的進步。

而本書收載更多的是有關醫學的典故資料。这些典故在人們閲讀熟知的基礎上，可進一步加工成新的成語典故，以便廣泛使用。這正是筆者編寫本書的用意所在。

本書編寫體例如下。每則典故分四個部分：首先是原文並標明出處；其二是簡要的注釋；其三是釋義，基本上是原文的語譯；其四是按語，僅做簡要的提示或必要的考證。

所有典故均按類編排，全書分醫史記聞、大醫精誠、養生健身、名醫軼事、名句箴言、醫鑒醫戒、辨證論治、奇方異案、情志之疾、雜説趣談、本草拾萃、諷喻世情、成語尋幽、傳説故事、破除迷信等十五個門類，分别編排在四個分册之中。第一分册含名醫軼事、情志之疾、本草拾萃、傳説故事四類，第二分册含醫史記聞、奇方異案、諷喻世情三類，第三分册含名句箴言、大醫精誠、辨證論治、養生健身四類，第四分册含醫鑒醫戒、雜説趣談、成語尋幽、破除迷信四類。每類之内，按選文的時代順序先後排列。以上分類，未必恰當，只是爲了方便閲讀而已。

本書的編寫經歷了較長的歲月，早在二十世紀八十年代初期我編寫《醫古文選讀》一書時，曾從古籍中收集到不少資料，便萌發了編寫此書的想法，並撰寫了一些片斷。之後，由於繁重的教學工作和衆多的寫作任務，此書的編寫工作時續時斷，我一旦收集到可用資料，便隨手寫上一篇或一段，裝入紙袋，以備後用。直到2003年，《河南中醫》雜志開設“醫林掌故”專欄，我便每期發一篇，連載至今，已達十三年之久。其間，在《大河健康報》等報刊上也發表一部分，先後刊載一百餘篇。不少讀者向我表示，希望能儘快出版此書，我也感到不能再拖延了。正好我已經退休，可以比較自由地掌握時間，於是全力投入了此書的編寫工作。當我整理完目録，望着一摞摞打印的書稿，感慨不已。近三十年時間，我無時不惦念着此事，星霜幾换，歲月悠悠，鷄聲燈影，甘苦自知。今天終於了却了心願，怎能不感到欣慰呢！

我在編寫本書的過程中，曾得到多人的幫助和支持。早在二十多年前，老友賈太誼主任醫師得知我要編寫此書，便積極爲我提供《本草綱目》中一些本草故事的資料，並親自撰寫了其中一部分初稿；我的研究生馬鴻祥、吴忠利及青年教師施淼等同志認真參與查找資料、校對書稿等繁瑣的工作；黄夏和尤佳二人幫助打印書稿並編排了全書的兩套目録；著名中醫文獻專家、北京中醫藥大學錢超塵教授和著名中醫文化學者、科普作家、中華中醫藥學會學術顧問温長路教授這兩位摯友，更是多次給予鼓勵和支持，並提出了許多建設性意見。還有不少同志給予幫助，不再一一列舉。正是大家的熱心幫助和支持，才使本書得以順利付梓。

該書内容在報刊連載以後，受到中醫界和文化界很多同志的關注和鼓勵，他们提出了許多建設性意見。河南中醫學院院長鄭玉玲教授高瞻遠矚，爲了向世界傳揚中醫藥文化，她親自策劃將此書譯成英文。兩年多來，在鄭院長及多位院系領導的大力支持下，由在瓦爾帕萊索大學任教的夏昀博士擔任總主譯，由河南中醫學院外語學院孫俊芳教授和朱文曉、蘇峰、穆海博、李曉婧、李蕾、李蘋、劉鴻等專家分别擔任各分册主譯，經過艱苦的努力而將其全部譯成英文。鄭院長還親自爲這部英漢對照版著作寫了序言。筆者謹在此向鄭院長和各位同志表示崇高的敬意和誠摯的感謝。同時，還要特别感謝本書的英文主審Nicholas Phillips、John Ruff、Evelyn Henry、Frank Phillips、王成至教授、孫俊芳教授等諸位女士和先生，是他們的辛勤工作才最終玉成此事。

由於本人水平所限，書中可能會有錯訛之處，懇請讀者批評指正。

許敬生

2014年12月31日

于河南中醫學院金水河畔問學齋

Preface

Among the tremendous amount of ancient medical works and other ancient works, there hid wisdom of renowned doctors and Traditional Chinese Medical knowledge. These stories are instructive and thought-provoking with inspiring enlightenment, wits, and delights. It's also helpful for learners to improve their classical Chinese level and competence of reading ancient medical classics. Yet, books on this topic are scarce. In the past years, I collected a lot of materials while reading ancient classics and have often been marveled at the profound TCM culture and the rich mine of Chinese language. Inspired to compile these works, I decide to sort out the medical literature hidden in ancient books and extract some new idioms and allusions to enrich the Chinese language repository.

Idioms and allusions are customized words and phrases long being used, repeatedly refined and polished to certain forms. They are quintessence of the language, normally melodious in phonetics, neat in structure, implicit in semantics, and vivid in feature. It is often through learning and using of the phrasal idioms that the modern people's memory of ancient Chinese is activated and kept alive.

It is well-known that the phrasal idioms come from ancient works, poetry, proses, slangs and proverbs. TCM, which is closely related to people's lives, is naturally one of the sources. This book includes some idioms which are directly traced to medical works, such as "the disease has attacked the vitals" "exhale the old and inhale the new" "apply medicine according to indications" "extreme joy begets sorrow" "beyond remedy" "a rolling stone gathers no moss, door pivot not cricket" "breaking arms three times makes a skilled doctor" etc. These idioms not only keep the medical implication, but also get wider social meaning by extending to other fields, to describe certain social phenomena. The mutual penetration of medicine and sociology in the usage of these idioms represents the development and popularization of TCM and the progress of the society.

The materials collected in this book are mainly from medical works. The author aims to refine and extract new phrasal idioms for people to use on the basis of reading and understanding them.

The structure of this book is like this: each story consists of four parts: original work and the source of the work, notes to the text, modern Chinese explanation, and the editor's notes, followed by English translation. The stories are compiled into fifteen categories in four volumes: the first volume has Anecdotes of Famous Doctors, Emotional Diseases, Finely Selected

Notes on Herbal Medicine, and Legends and Stories; the second volume consists of Records of Medical History, Unusual Cases and Unconventional Treatments, and Allegories Related to Medical Treatments; the third volume includes Illuminating Quotes and Maxims, Doctors of Utmost Medical Excellence and Ethics, Differential Diagnosis and Treatment, Guarding Life and Cultivating Health; the fourth volume is made up of Drawing Lessons from Past Medical Cases, Miscellaneous Thoughts and Anecdotes, Origins of Chinese Idioms Relevant to Medicine, and Medical Explanations for Supernatural Beings and Phenomena. Every category is arranged in time sequence. The division of the categories is not necessarily appropriate, but just for the convenience of the readers. The bibliography and index of Pinyin are provided at the end of the book for the readers to refer to.

It took me many years to finish the book. While I was compiling the textbook *Selected Readings of Ancient Chinese Medical Literature* I collected a lot of classic resources and came up the idea of compiling this book and started with some segments. Since then, the work on the book was on again off again for a while because of the heavy workload and writing commitments. But when I came across some useful resources, I noted them down and put them into my pocket for future use. It was not until 2003, when the Journal of *Henan Traditional Chinese Medicine* started the new column "medical quotations and allusions" that my collections were published, one article at an issue, for thirteen years. More than 100 of these articles were published in *Dahe Health News* at the same time. Many readers expected me to publish this book as soon as possible, and I also feel I shouldn't delay the work anymore. Then I spared no efforts into this book since I had more time at my disposal at my retirement. After I put the contents in order and looked at the pile of the printed manuscript in front, all sorts of feelings welled up in my mind. For thirty years I had been thinking of this book. For years, in long nights, in early dawn, in frosty winter and hot summer days, I had been tasting the joy and frustration of writing this book. Now finally my wish was fulfilled, how could I not feel joy and relief?

Many people contributed to the compiling of the book. As early as more than twenty years ago, when my old friend Jia Taiyi got to know that I was working on this book, he provided some herbal stories from the book *Compendium of Materia Medica* and even wrote part of it; My postgraduate students Ma Hongxiang, Wu Zhongli and a young teacher Shi Miao got involved in the tedious task of looking up the references and proofreading. Huang Xia and You Jia helped with typing and printing of the manuscripts and worked with the two sets of contents of the book. My dear friends Qian Chaochen, a renowned TCM literature expert and professor in Beijing University of TCM, and Wen Changlu, a famous scholar in TCM culture, popular science writer and adviser of China Association of Chinese Medicine provided me continuous encouragement and support with constructive suggestions. Many other people contributed to this work but it was impossible for me to acknowledge them all here. It was owing to all these people's help and support that this book was able to be published finally.

The book has received many people's attention in the field of TCM and culture since it came out as a serial. Many people gave me their encouragement and constructive suggestions. Zheng Yuling, the president of Henan University of TCM is far-sighted to plan out the translation of the book in order to publicize the TCM culture to the world. In the past two years, with the support of President Zheng and other university leaders, the translation work has been successfully done with Dr. Xia Yun as the main translator, Sun Junfang, Zhu Wenxiao, Su Feng, Mu Haibo, Li Xiaojing, Li Lei, Li Ping, and Liu Hong as the translators-in-chief for the four volumes. President Zheng even wrote the preface for the book. I want to present my high respect and heart-felt thanks to these people. At the same time, I owe my gratitude to the English language proofreaders Nicholas Phillips, John Ruff, Evelyn Henry, Frank Phillips, Professor Wang Chengzhi, Professor Sun Junfang, etc. for their contribution. Without their hard work, it would have been impossible to finish the book.

With My limitation, it will be hard to avoid errors and mistakes in this book. So I sincerely invite my dear readers for your advice and corrections.

Xu Jingsheng

December 31, 2014

In Wenxue Study, Henan University of TCM by Jinshui River

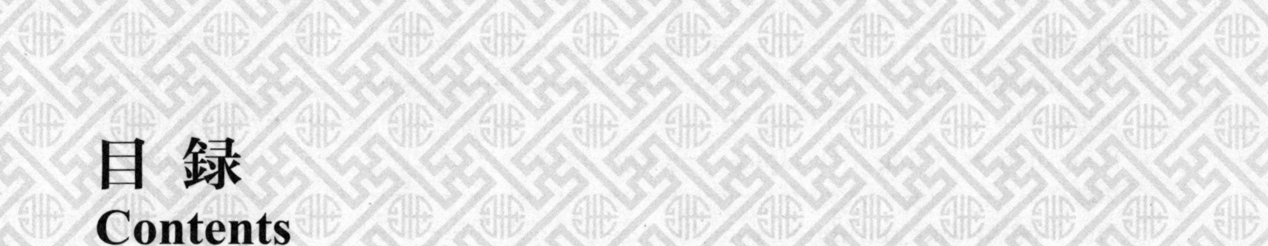

目録
Contents

情志之疾 Emotional Diseases……057

本草拾萃 Finely Selected Notes on Herbal Medicine······ 100

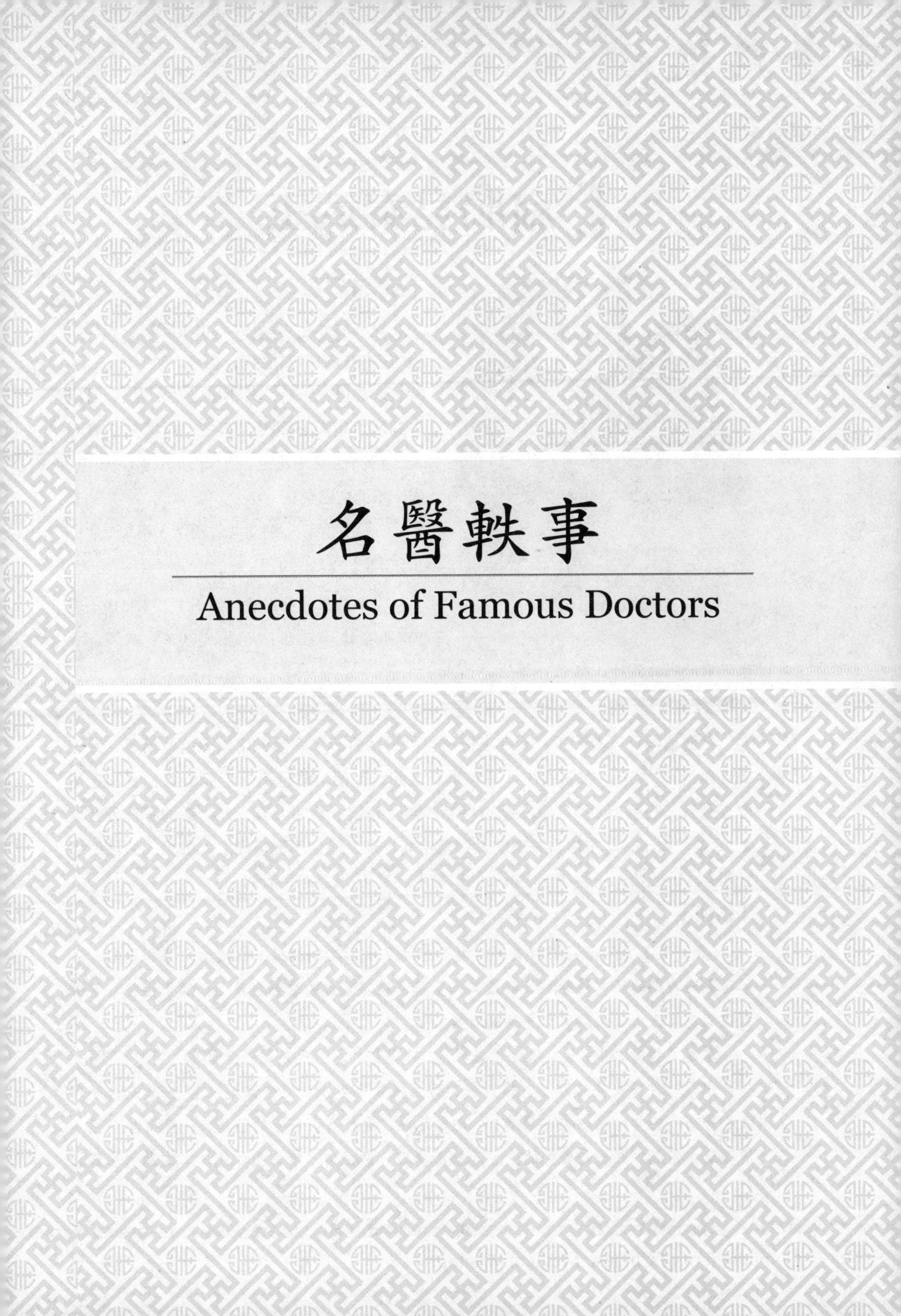

名醫軼事

Anecdotes of Famous Doctors

【扁鵲見秦武王】

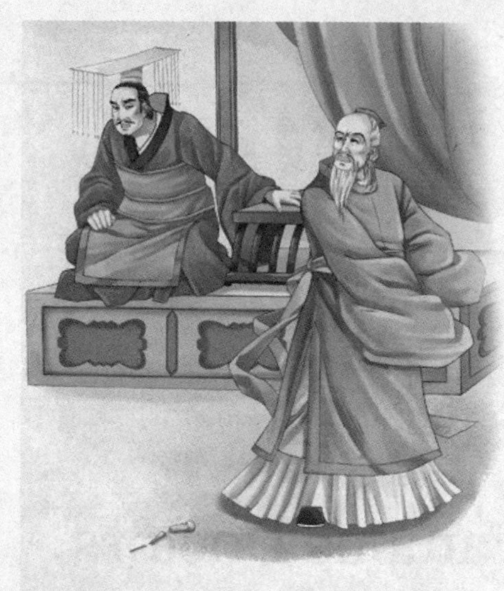

【原文】

醫扁鵲見秦武王[1]。武王示之病，扁鵲請除[2]。左右曰："君之病，在耳之前，目之下，除之未必已也，將使耳不聰，目不明。"君以告扁鵲。扁鵲怒而投其石[3]："君與知之者謀之，而與不知之者敗之。使[4]此知[5]秦國之政也，則一舉而亡國矣！"

（選自西漢 · 劉向《戰國策 · 秦策二》）

【注釋】

①秦武王：戰國時秦國國君，前310—前307年在位。② 除：治療。 ③石：砭石。古代用來治病的石針。④使：假使。⑤知：主管。

【釋義】

名醫扁鵲拜見秦武王。秦武王把自己的病情告訴了扁鵲，扁鵲願給他治療。武王的近臣說："大王，您的病在耳朵和眼睛之間，即使治療也不一定能治愈，說不定還會耳朵聾、眼睛不明。"武王把這些話告訴了扁鵲。扁鵲大怒，把治病的石針丟在地上，說："大王，您跟懂得醫理的人商量治病，却又聽信不懂醫理之人的話。假使這樣管理秦國的政治，只要在一次重大的舉動上遲疑不決，秦國就會滅亡！"

【按語】

《戰國策》是一部國別體史書，主要記述了戰國時期縱橫家的政治主張和策略，展示了戰國時期的歷史特點和社會風貌，是研究戰國歷史的重要典籍。西漢末由著名學者劉向編定爲三十三篇，書名亦爲劉向所擬定。

醫學是精微之事，只有用心精微者，方可與言之。明代大醫張介賓在《病家兩要説》一文中，一再强調要忌浮言，擇真醫，而且任醫要專一。他感慨地説："夫如是，是醫之于醫尚不能知，而矧夫非醫者！"意思是説，對於高明醫生的治法，一般醫生尚且不能理解，何況那些不是醫生的人呢。推而廣之，做任何事情都是如此。本文通過扁鵲爲秦武王診病的故事，告誡治國者要“與知之者謀之”，不要“與不知之者敗之”，以免貽誤國家。

Bian Que[1] Met with King Wu of Qin[2]

The famous doctor Bian Que paid a formal visit to King Wu of Qin. The king described his symptoms and Bian Que was going to treat him. However, the king's courtiers said, "My Lord, where you feel the discomfort lies between your ears and eyes. Even if you agree to receive the treatment, it probably would not work. What's worse, you might become deaf and lose your eyesight." The king told these words to Bian Que. After hearing that, Bian Que angrily dropped the healing stone and needles onto the ground and said: "Your Majesty, you consulted a medical professional about your disease, but then readily believed people without any medical knowledge. How could that ever work? Suppose you are governing the State of Qin with such a method, the kingdom would be destroyed if you hesitate to make an important decision!"

From *Strategies of the Warring States*[3].

Notes:

1. Bian Que (扁鵲 ca. 700 BCE): aka Bian Qiao, was the earliest known Chinese physician. His real name was said to be Qin Yueren (秦越人).

2. King Wu of Qin (秦武王 310–307 BCE): He is the ruler of the Qin State (秦 , 221–207 BCE) from the Warring States Period of Chinese history.

3. *Strategies of the Warring States* (《戰國策》Zhanguo Ce): It is a renowned ancient Chinese historical work and compilation of sporadic materials on the Warring States period compiled between the 3rd to 1st centuries BCE. It is an important text of the Warring States Period as it accounts the strategies and political views of the School of Diplomacy and reveals the historical and social characteristics of the period.

Editor's Note:

This excerpt recorded that Bian Que treated the disease of King Wu of Qin, which serves as a warning to rulers and governors that they should only talk about important matters with those who truly understand them.

【扁鵲隨俗爲變】

【原文】

扁鵲名聞天下。過邯鄲，聞貴[①]婦人，即爲帶下醫[②]；過雒陽[③]，聞周人愛老人，即爲耳目痹醫[④]；來入咸陽，聞秦人愛小兒，即爲小兒醫。隨俗爲[⑤]變。

（選自西漢・司馬遷《史記・扁鵲倉公列傳》）

【注釋】

①貴：重視、尊重。②帶下醫：婦科醫生。帶下，帶脈以下。一般婦科病帶證居多，故名。③雒（luò 洛）陽：即洛陽，東周王都所在地。雒，同“洛”。④耳目痹醫：治耳、目、痹病的醫生，即專治老年病的醫生。⑤爲：而。連詞。

【釋義】

扁鵲的名聲傳遍天下。到邯鄲，聽説當地尊重婦女，就做婦科醫生。到洛陽，聽説周都之人敬愛老人，就做專治耳、目、痹疾的老年病醫生；來到咸陽，聽説秦地之人疼愛兒童，就做兒科醫生。隨着各地的習俗而改變行醫的科別。

【按語】

司馬遷（約前145或前135—？），是中國古代偉大的史學家、文學家、思想家。被後世尊稱爲“史聖”。他最大的貢獻是創作了中國第一部紀傳體通史《史記》，記載了上自黄帝，下至漢武帝長達三千多年的歷史。

《史記・扁鵲倉公列傳》是中國醫學史上第一篇醫家傳記。

扁鵲能“隨俗爲變”，説明他的醫術既精當又全面，這也是適應社會的需要，因而深受人民的愛戴。

Bian Que Adjusting His Practice According to Local Needs

Bian Que was quite famous throughout the country, and was adaptable in his practice. When Bian Que arrived at Handan and heard that the local people respected women, he would serve as a gynecologist. When he arrived at Luoyang and heard that people in the capital of Zhou respected the elderly, he would serve as a geriatrician to treat problems with ears, eyes and bidisease. When he arrived at Xianyang and heard that people in that region of Qin loved children dearly, he would serve as a pediatrician. His medical specialty changed based on local customs and needs.

From *Records of the Grand Historian*[1].

Notes:

1. *Records of the Grand Historian* (《史記》Shiji) : Written from 109 BCE to 91 BCE, it was a masterpiece of historical work by Sima Qian[2], in which he recounted Chinese history from the time of the Yellow Emperor until his own time. (The Yellow Emperor, was the first ruler whom Sima Qian considered sufficiently established as historical to appear in the Records.)

2. Sima Qian: (司馬遷，ca. 145 BCE or 135 BCE – ?) was a Chinese historian of Han Dynasty. He won the name of "The father of Chinese historiography" for his work, the *Records of the Grand Historian*, a history of China to his time written in the biographical style. Although he worked as the Imperial Astronomer (太 史 令) , later generations refer to him as the Grand Historian (太史公) for his monumental work.

Editor's Note:

Bian Que adapted to the demand of the society by conforming to the local customs and serving local needs, and thus was deeply trusted and loved by people. This excerpt also reflects his supreme and comprehensive medical skills.

【扁鵲診趙簡子疾】

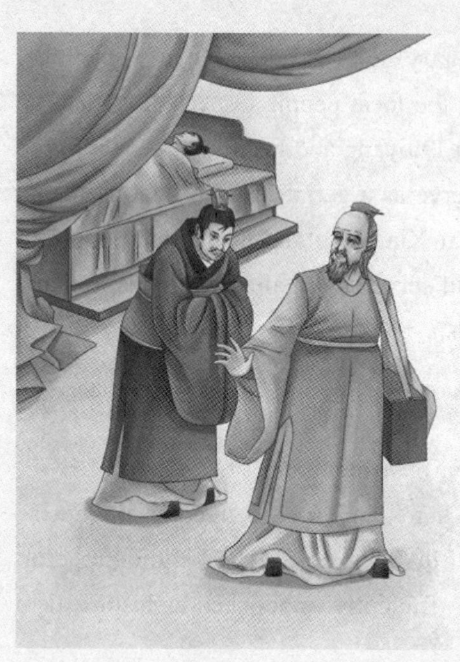

【原文】

當晉昭公[①]時，諸大夫强而公族[②]弱，趙簡子[③]爲大夫，專[④]國事。簡子疾，五日不知人，大夫皆懼，于是召扁鵲。扁鵲入，視病，出，董安于[⑤]問扁鵲，扁鵲曰："血脈治[⑥]也，而[⑦]何怪！昔秦穆公[⑧]嘗如此，七日而寤。……今主君之病與之同，不出三日必間[⑨]，間必有言也。"居二日半，簡子寤。

（選自西漢 · 司馬遷《史記 · 扁鵲倉公列傳》）

【注釋】

①晉昭公：春秋時晉國國君。姓姬名夷，在位六年（前531—前526）。②公族：又稱"公姓"。這裏指晉國國君的家族。③趙簡子：趙鞅，亦稱趙孟，簡子是謚號。④專：專擅，獨掌。⑤董安于：趙簡子的家臣。⑥治：正常。⑦而：你，代詞。⑧秦穆公：春秋時秦國國君，姓嬴，名任好。前659—前621年在位。⑨間（jiàn 見）：病愈。

【釋義】

在晉昭公的時候，衆大夫的勢力强大，而國君家族的勢力弱小。趙簡子做大夫，獨攬國家政事。趙簡子生病，五天不省人事，大夫都很害怕，于是召見扁鵲診治。扁鵲進入宫廷，診察趙簡子的病，然后走出來。趙簡子家臣董安于向扁鵲詢問，扁鵲回答説："血脈正常，你驚怪什麼呢！從前秦穆公也曾經像這樣，七日就醒過來了。現在您主人的病跟秦穆公相同，不超過三日一定痊愈。"過了二日半，趙簡子果真醒過來了。

【按語】

通過記述扁鵲給趙簡子診病的故事，說明扁鵲不僅精于切脈，診斷準確，而且歷史知識豐富。

Bian Que Examining Zhao Jianzi

During the reign of King Zhao of Jin[1], ministers with the rank of Dafu[2] were quite powerful while the royalty was often weak. Zhao Jianzi, as a Dafu, dominated the political affairs of the Jin State. Once he was ill and had fallen unconscious for five days. Other officials was scared and called in Bian Que to treat him. Bian Que entered the palace, examined Zhao's disease and then came out. Zhao's retainer Dong Anyu came to inquire him about the condition. Bian Que answered, "His blood circulation is normal. Why are you making a fuss about it? The former Duke Mu of Qin[3] had the same symptoms. He woke up and recovered in seven days. Now that your masters' disease is quite similar to his, he'll certainly recover within three days." After two days and a half, Zhao Jianzi really was back to his normal himself.

From *Records of the Grand Historian*.

Notes:

1. King Zhao of Jin (晉昭公 died 526 BCE): He was from 531 BCE to 526 BCE the ruler of the Jin State , a major power during the Spring and Autumn Period of ancient China.

2. Dafu (大夫): It is a senior official rank in ancient China.

3. Duke Mu of Qin (秦穆公 , died in 621 BCE): He reigned from 659 BCE to 621 BCE as the fourteenth ruler of the Qin State .

Editor's Note:

Bian Que was not only good at pulse-taking and making diagnosis, but also knowledgeable in history.

【倉公望診】

【原文】

齊王黃姬[1]兄黃長卿家有酒召客，召臣意。諸客坐，未上食。臣意望見王后弟宋建，告曰："君有病，往[2]四五日；君要[3]脅痛，不可俯仰，又不得小溲。不亟治，病即入濡腎[4]。及其未舍五藏，急治之。病方今客腎濡[5]，此所謂腎痹[6]也。"宋建曰："然。建故[7]有要脊痛。往四五日，天雨，黃氏諸倩見建家京下[8]方石，即弄之，建亦欲效之，效之不能起[9]，即復置之。暮，要脊痛，不得溺[10]，至今不愈。"建病得之好持重[11]。所以知建病者，臣意見其色，太陽色乾[12]，腎部上及界要以下者枯四分所[13]，故以往四五日知其發也。臣意即爲柔湯[14]使服之，十八日所而病愈。

（選自西漢 · 司馬遷《史記 · 扁鵲倉公列傳》）

【注釋】

①姬：帝王之妃嬪。②往：以往，過去。③要：同"腰"，下同。④濡腎：染及腎臟。濡，浸染。⑤客腎濡：病正侵入腎臟，因而影響小便。客，寄居，指病邪自外侵入。⑥腎痹：古病名。指腎氣閉塞不通。⑦故：通"固"，確實。⑧倩：女婿。京下：糧倉下邊。京，穀倉。⑨起：舉起。⑩溺：通"尿"。⑪好持重：喜歡拿舉重物。⑫太陽色乾：太陽部位的面色乾枯。其位在眼眶外後方，即顳顬（niè rú）。一說，太陽似爲"大腸"，大腸經的色診部位在面部中央。⑬上及界：指腎部向上直到與太陽部位的交界處。要（腰）以下：指腎部下端。所：許，左右。⑭柔湯：溫補之湯劑。與"剛劑"相對。

【釋義】

齊王姓黃的妃子之兄黃長卿家有酒會客，也邀請我，與衆客就座，尚未上食。我看見了王后之弟宋建，就告訴他說："您有病，前四五天，您的腰脅痛得不能俯仰，小便又不通暢。不趕快治療，病就要向內浸染腎臟。應趁它未入侵五臟時趕快治療。今病將侵入腎而影響小便，這就是所說的腎痹之病。"宋建說："對。我確實有腰脊痛。前四五天，天下着雨，黃家衆女婿看到我家糧倉下面有塊方石，就搬弄它，我也想模仿他們，學他們搬弄方石，但不能舉起，就又放下它。傍晚時，腰脊痛，不能小便，到如今也不見好。"宋建的病從喜好持取重物而得。我知道宋建患病的原因，是望見他的面色，在太陽部位顏色乾枯，臀部向上至交界處和腰臀以下部位的面色乾枯四分左右。所以又知道他發病在前四五天。我立即製作温補的湯藥使他服下，十八天左右病就好了。

【按語】

倉公淳于意通過望面色，準確地診斷了宋建的腎痹病，並用“柔湯”治愈之。爲後人留下了一個典型病例。

Diagnosis by Inspection

Huang Changqing, the brother of an imperial concubine, entertained guests one day, and I was among the invited. Before meal was served, seated with other guests, I saw the queen's brother Song Jian and told him, "You are not well. Since four to five days ago, you have not been able to bend or stretch due to the pain around your waist and ribs. In addition, you cannot urinate as normal. If you do not receive a treatment soon, the disease would affect your kidney, which is the so-called renal obstruction. You should treat it before it attacks the five internal organs." Song Jian said, "Yes, my waist and spine were painful indeed. Four to five days ago, when it was raining, Huang's sons-in-law saw a stone in my granary and lifted it. I tried to do the same but could not, so I put it down. Later I began to feel the pain in waist and spine. I couldn't piss and haven't been treated up to now." Song Jian's disease resulted from his attempt to hold heavy things. I found this from his dull complexion at the temple and a little bit of glow on cheeks and chins, which reflected problems with waist and kidney. From this, I became aware that he fell ill four to five days ago. Then I immediately made the warmly invigorating prescribed medicine for him to take. Eighteen days later, his illness fully recovered.

From *Records of the Grand Historian*.

Editor's Note:

This excerpt is a classic case of diagnosis in medical history. Chunyu Yi correctly diagnosed Song Jian's renal obstruction and cured him by "Routang" , a type of TCM formula.

【蒜齏治咽塞】

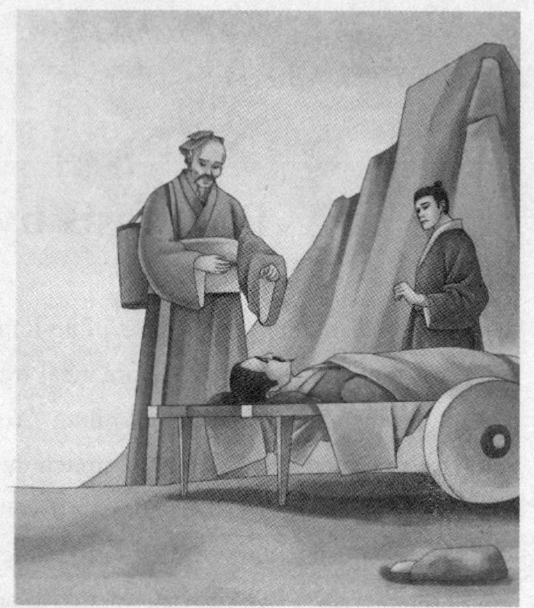

【原文】

佗行道，見一人病咽塞[1]，嗜食而不得下。家人車載欲往就醫。佗聞其呻吟，駐車[2]往視，語之曰："向[3]來道邊有賣餠家，蒜齏大酢[4]，從取三升飲之，病自當去。"即如佗言，立吐虵[5]一枚，縣[6]車邊，欲造佗。佗尚未還，小兒戲門前，逆見[7]，自相謂[8]曰："似逢我公[9]，車邊病[10]是也。"疾者前入坐，見佗北壁縣此虵輩約以十數[11]。

（選自西晉 · 陳壽《三國志 · 華佗傳》）

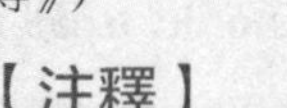

【注釋】

①咽塞：咽喉阻塞。②駐車：停下車。③向：方才。④蒜齏：蒜汁。大酢：很酸。酢，同"醋"；（古）酸。⑤虵："蛇"的異體字。此指蛔蟲一類的寄生蟲。⑥縣："懸"的古字。 ⑦逆見：迎面看到。 ⑧自相謂：自己對自己說，即自言自語。相，稱代性副詞。 ⑨公：此指父親。 ⑩車邊病：指車邊掛着的寄生蟲。⑪十數：即數十條。

【釋義】

華佗在路上行走，看見一人患咽部阻塞，想進食可是不能咽下，他的家人用車子拉着他前往就醫。華佗聽到病人的呻吟，把車子停下前往診視，告訴病人說："剛才過來的路邊有賣餠的人，他的蒜汁非常酸，向他求取三升飲服，病自然就會好。"病人按華佗所說的去做，立刻吐出一條蛇一樣的寄生蟲，便把它懸掛在車邊，打算到華佗家去。華佗還没有回來，他的小兒在門前戲玩，迎面見到來人，就自言自語地說："好像遇到了我的父親，車邊掛的病物就是證明。"病人前往進屋入座，看見華佗家中北牆上掛着這一類寄生蟲，大約有幾十條。

【按語】

陳壽（233—297）西晉史學家，著有《三國志》。《三國志》共六十五卷，分魏、蜀、吴三志。

從這段記載可以看出，飲服足量蒜汁治療咽塞病，催吐腹中寄生蟲，是華佗的成功經驗。他家中北牆上掛的幾十條蛇一樣的寄生蟲，就是有力的證明。

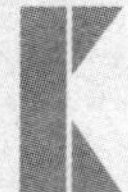

Mashed Garlic for Obstruction in the Throat

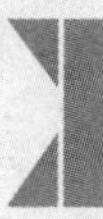

Hua Tuo once met a person suffering from obstruction in the throat. The patient wanted to eat but could not swallow, thus was sent to the doctor with a handcart by his family members. Hua Tuo heard the patient moaning, stopped the handcart to examine and told the patient, "There's a person selling pancakes on the roadside. His mashed garlic is quite sour. You should ask him for three sheng (an ancient volume unit, which is approximately equal to 200mL). Take it and then you will recover." The patient did as what Hua Tuo told him, and spit out a snake-like parasite. He hanged the parasite beside the cart and went to Hua Tuo's home to thank him. Hua Tuo was not home yet. His little son was playing in front of the door. Seeing the visiter, the child said to himself, "Seems that he's met my father. The parasite is the evidence." The patient entered Hua Tuo's house and found dozens of such kind of parasites hung on the northern wall.

From *History of the Three Kingdoms*[1].

Notes:

1. *History of the Three Kingdoms* (《三國志》Sanguozhi): It is a Chinese historical text that covers the history of the Eastern Han Dynasty and the Three Kingdoms Period. It is widely regarded as the official and authoritative historical text for that period. Written by Chen Shou in the 3rd century, the work combines the accounts of the rival states of Wei, Shu and Wu in the Three Kingdoms period into a single text. *History of the Three Kingdoms* provided the basis for the historical novel *Romance of the Three Kingdoms* (《三國演義》Sanguo Yanyi), written by Luo Guanzhong in the 14th century.

Editor's Note:

Hua Tuo successfully treated throat obstruction more than once and purged abdominal parasites by mashed garlic. Parasites hung on his wall were powerful evidence.

【華佗爲頓子獻診病】

【原文】

故督郵[①]頓子獻得病已差，詣佗視脈，曰："尚虛，未得復，勿爲勞事[②]，御内即死。臨死，當吐舌數寸。"其妻聞其病除，從百餘里來省之，止宿交接，中間[③]三日發病，一如佗言。

（選自西晉 · 陳壽《三國志 · 華佗傳》）

【注釋】

①故：原來的。督郵：官名。漢置。爲郡守佐吏，掌督察糾舉所領縣違法之事。②勞事：房勞之事。下文"御内""交接"，義同此。③間：間隔。

【釋義】

原督郵頓子獻患病已經好了，來請華佗診察脈象，華佗說："你的身體還很虛弱，没有完全康復，不要行房事，如果行房事就要死去。臨死的時候會吐出幾寸長舌。"他的妻子聽說他的病已經好了，就從一百多里外來看望他，夜裏歇息時夫妻行房事，相隔三天後頓子獻發病，完全像華佗預言的那樣。

【按語】

這段記載説明，有些病在未康復之前，是須要禁房事的，如若不禁，將會導致嚴重的後果。頓子獻不聽華佗的勸告，導致病發而死，就是一個例證。

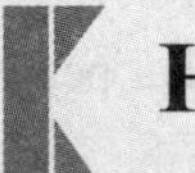

Hua Tuo Warned Dun Zixian

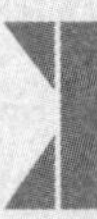

A former official Dun Zixian recovered from a disease and asked Hua Tuo to examine his pulse. Hua Tuo said, "You are still weak and not yet completely recovered. Do avoid sexual intercourse. If not, you will die with your tongue sticking out for several cun." Hearing that he had recovered, his wife came to visit him from more than one hundred li away. They had sex during the night. Three days later, Dun Zixian's disease was back again, and he died just as Hua had described.

From *History of the Three Kingdoms*.

Editor's Note:

Patients should avoid sexual intercourse if they have not yet recovered. Otherwise, some serious consequences may occur. Dun Zixian ignored the advice of Hua Tuo and then died of the recurrent disease. This excerpt is an example.

【四十眉落】

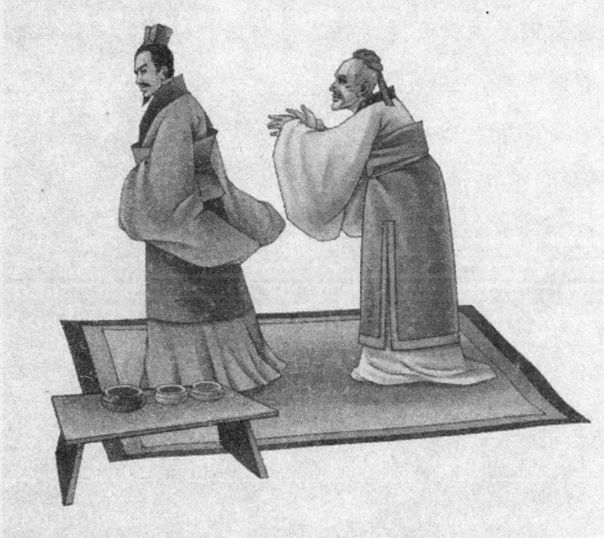

【原文】

仲景見侍中①王仲宣②，時年二十餘，謂曰："君有病，四十當眉落，眉落半年而死。"令服五石湯③可免。仲宣嫌其言忤④，受湯勿服。居三日，見仲宣，謂曰："服湯否？"曰："已服。"仲景曰："色候固非服湯之診，君何輕命也！"仲宣猶不言。後二十年果眉落，後一百八十七日而死，終如其言。

（選自晉・皇甫謐《針灸甲乙經・序》）

【注釋】

①侍中：漢代侍從皇帝左右，出入宮廷的官。②王仲宣：名粲（177—217），山陽高平（今山東鄒縣）人。建安七子之一。③五石湯：由陽起石、鐘乳石、靈磁石、空青石、金剛石等組成。④忤：逆耳。

【釋義】

張仲景遇見侍中王仲宣，當時仲宣只有二十多歲，仲景對他說："你有病，到四十歲眉毛會脱落，眉脱半年之後就將死亡。"並叫他服五石湯，說可以治愈此病，免除死亡。王仲宣嫌張仲景的話逆耳不恭，接受藥方却不服藥。過了三天，張仲景又見到王仲宣，問他説："湯藥服了没有？"仲宣回答説："已經服過了。"張仲景説："從您的面色證候來看，根本不像服過五石湯的樣子，您爲什麼這樣輕視自己的生命呢？"王仲宣仍是避而不答。二十年後，仲宣的眉毛果然脱落，眉落後一百八十七天便死去了，終於像張仲景預言的那樣。

【按語】

皇甫謐（214—282），魏晉著名學者、醫學家。字士安，幼名静，自號玄晏先生，安定朝那（今寧夏固原東南，一説甘肅靈台境内）人。中年患風痹症，後專心攻讀醫書，撰成《黄帝三部針灸甲乙經》，總結了晉代以前的針灸成就，是現存最早的針灸學專著。原書根據天干編次，故命名爲《針灸甲乙經》。此外，還著有《帝王世紀》《玄晏春秋》等多種史學著作。

仲景（150—219），東漢傑出的醫學家張仲景。著《傷寒雜病論》一書，集漢以前醫學之大成，後人奉其爲醫方之祖，尊爲醫聖。

王仲宣，名粲（177—217），漢末文學家，建安七子之一。

仲景望診王仲宣，同越人入虢之診、望齊侯之色一樣，皆謂之神奇。雖説不免有誇張的色彩，但它反映了人們對名醫高超的望診技術的推崇。而這種望診技術，正是中醫的奥妙所在。這則故事還啓示人們，要見微知著，爲了避免疾病的發生，應當接受真醫的良言相勸，哪怕有些逆耳。假若王仲宣不"嫌其言忤"，服用了仲景所給之藥，就不會出現"眉落半年而死"的悲劇。

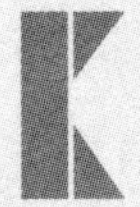

Eyebrows Shed at Forty Years Old

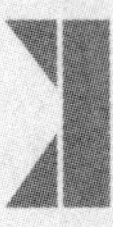

Zhang Zhongjing[1] met a high official, Wang Zhongxuan[2], who was only in his twenties then. Zhongjing told him, "You've got a disease. In your forties, your eyebrows will fall and half a year later you will die." He prescribed Five Stone Decoction[3] to treat Wang's disease and tried to save him from death. Wang found Zhang Zhongjing's words offensive, so he accepted the prescription but did not take it. Three days later, Zhang

Zhongjing met Wang Zhongxuan again and asked, "Have you taken the decoction?" Zhongxuan lied to him by saying yes. Zhang Zhongjing said, "Judging from your complexion and symptoms, you have not taken the decoction. Why do you take your own life so lightly?" Wang Zhongxuan still refused to do what Zhang suggested. Twenty years later, Zhongxuan's eyebrows really started to shed and died after 187 days, which confirmed Zhang Zhongjing's prediction.

From *Canon of Acupuncture and Moxibustion*.

Notes:

1. Zhang Zhongjing (張仲景 ac.2 to 3 century): With the formal name Zhang Ji (張機), he was a Han Dynasty physician and one of the most eminent Chinese physicians in history.

2. Wang Zhongxuan (王仲宣) : He was also known as Wang Can (王粲，177–217), was a Chinese politician, scholar and poet during the late Han Dynasty. He contributed greatly to the establishment of laws and standards for the Wei State of the Three Kingdoms period. For his literary achievement, Wang Can was ranked among the "Seven Scholars of Jian'an" (建安七子).

3. Five Stone Decoction (五石湯 Wushi Tang) : The decoction was the mixture of actinolite, stalactite, magnetitum, hollow azurite and diamond, etc.

Editor's Note:

Though a little exaggerated, the story reflects people's admiration of famous doctors' supreme diagnosis skills. The inspection examination showed the magic of the traditional Chinese medicine. The story also urges people to accept the advice of good doctors, which might be unpleasant to the ears. Suppose Wang Zhongxuan had taken Zhongjing's prescription, the tragedy could have been prevented.

【謐母泣教】

【原文】

皇甫謐，字士安，幼名静，安定朝那人①，漢太尉嵩②之曾孫也。出後叔父③，徙居新安④。年二十，不好學，游蕩無度，或以爲癡。嘗得瓜果，輒進所後叔母任氏。任氏曰："《孝經》云：'三牲⑤之養，猶爲不孝。'汝今年餘二十，目不存教，心不入道，無以慰我。"因嘆曰："昔孟母三徙⑥以成仁，曾父烹豕⑦以存教，豈我居不卜⑧鄰，教有所闕⑨？何爾魯鈍之甚也！修身篤學⑩，自汝得之，於我何有？"因對之流涕。謐乃感激⑪，就鄉人席坦受書，勤力不怠。居貧，躬自稼穡⑫，帶經而農，遂博綜典籍百家之言。

（選自《晉書・皇甫謐傳》）

【注釋】

①安定：郡名。漢置。朝（zhū 朱）那：縣名。②太尉嵩：東漢靈帝時太尉皇甫嵩。太尉，漢時中央最高軍事長官。③出後叔父：過繼給叔父。出後，猶"出繼"，即過繼。④徙：遷居。新安：郡名。漢丹陽郡地，三國吴分置新都郡，晉太康元年（280年）改名新安郡。在今浙江省淳安西。一說是今河南省新安縣。⑤三牲：牛、羊、猪。《孝經・紀孝行章》："事親者，居上不驕，爲下不亂，在醜（衆）不争，……三者不除，雖日用三牲之養，猶爲不孝。"⑥孟母三徙：相傳孟軻年幼時，所居環境不好，孟母爲教育孟軻，三次遷居。事見《列女傳・母儀》和趙岐《孟子題辭》。後喻母教之德。⑦曾父烹豕（shǐ 史）：曾參妻攜子到市場，其子啼哭，母親説回家後爲子殺猪。回家後，曾子將殺猪，其妻説與兒戲言，曾參認爲不能失信於子，終殺猪以取信。事見《韓非子・外儲説左上》。⑧卜：選擇。⑨闕：通"缺"。⑩篤學：專心學習。⑪ 感激：感動奮發。⑫躬自稼穡：躬，親自。稼穡，種莊稼、幹農活。

【釋義】

皇甫謐，表字士安，幼年時名静，安定郡朝那縣人，是漢太尉皇甫嵩的曾孫。過繼給叔父做兒子，遷居到新安郡。年紀已二十歲，仍不愛學習，放蕩不羈，有人認爲他癡呆。有一次得了瓜果，來進獻給叔母任氏。任氏説："《孝經》中説：'即使用三牲奉養，仍然是不孝。'你現在二十多歲了，眼中不存教化，心中不入大道，没有什麽東西可以安慰我的。”於是感嘆地說：“從前孟子的母親三次遷居以便培養孟子，曾參特意殺猪以便取信兒子，難道是我居處没選擇好鄰居，教育有什麽失誤嗎？爲什麽你魯莽愚鈍得如此嚴重呢！修身勤學，自然是你自己得到益處，對我來説有什麽呢？”於是對着他痛哭流涕。皇甫謐終於感動激發，跟從同鄉人席坦學習經書，勤奮努力，從不懈怠。他生活清貧，親身耕種，常常帶着經書而做農活，於是廣泛學習經典古籍和百家著作。

【按語】

《晉書》共一百三十卷，記載了從司馬懿開始到晉恭帝元熙二年爲止，包括西晉和東晉的歷史，並用“載記”的形式兼述了十六國割據政權的興亡。《晉書》爲二十四史之一，編者共二十一人，主持監修者爲房玄齡等。房玄齡（579—648），唐代初年名臣，名喬，字玄齡，以字行於世。唐代齊州臨淄（今山東淄博）人。

歷史上有成就的人，不管是年少早慧，還是大器晚成，良好的家教往往起着重要的作用。“孟母三遷”是如此，“曾父烹豕”是如此，“謐母泣教”更是如此。“年二十，不好學，游蕩無度”的青年皇甫謐，正是在養母情真意切流涕教誨的感召下，才幡然悔悟的。在爾後的歲月里，他樹立了“高尚之志”，“勤力不怠，手不輟卷”，最終成爲舉世聞名的文學家、史學家和醫學家。真應了那句俗話：浪子回頭金不换。

The Mother Who Guided Her Son in Tears

Huangfu Mi[1], with a courtesy name Shi'an, was the great-grandson of the Grand Commandant Huangfu Song in the Han Dynasty. His uncle adopted him, and then moved to Xin'an County. Until he was twenty years old, he had not focused on study, squandering his time all day long. People thought him worthless. Once he brought some fruits to visit his foster mother Ren. Ren said, “According to *Classic of Filial Piety* [2], dedicating even the most exquisite gifts or food does not make one filial. You've been twenty years old, but are still not versed in classics. Nothing else could comfort me.” She then wept, saying, “In the past, the mother of Mencius moved three times to pick the best location for him to grow up, and Zeng Shen killed the pig to teach his son a lesson about keeping one's promise. Hadn't I chosen a good neighbor or have I made any mistake in education? Why have you been so slack? Self-cultivation and diligence naturally benefit you. What can I do to motivate you to study?" Deeply moved and inspired, Huangfu Mi studied the classics with a tutor diligently and never slackened. He lived in poverty, worked on a farm, and enriched himself with classics. He became a highly regarded scholar.

From *The Book of the Jin Dynasty* [3].

Notes:

1. Huangfu Mi (皇甫謐 215–282): He was a Chinese scholar and physician during the late Han Dynasty. He compiled the *Canon of Acupuncture and Moxibustion* , a collection of various texts on acupuncture written in earlier periods. This book of 12 volumes further divided into 128 chapters was one of the earliest systematic works on acupuncture and moxibustion, and it proved to be one of the most influential. Huangfu Mi also compiled 10 books in a series called *Records of Emperors and Kings* (《帝王世紀》 Diwang Shiji).

2. *Classic of Filial Piety* (《孝經》 Xiaojing): It is a Confucian classic treatise giving advice on filial piety, that is, how to behave towards one's parents and senior relatives with propriety.

3. *The Book of the Jin Dynasty* (《晉書》 Jinshu): It is an official Chinese historical text covering the history of the Jin Dynasty. It was compiled by a number of scholar-officials commissioned by the imperial court of the Tang Dynasty, drawing mostly from official documents left from earlier archives. A few essays in volumes 1, 3, 54 and 80 were composed by Emperor Taizong of Tang himself. The contents of *The Book of the Jin Dynasty*, however, included not only the history of the Jin Dynasty, but also that of the Sixteen Kingdoms period, which was concurrent with the Eastern Jin Dynasty.

Editor's Note:

Good family education greatly contributes to the success of many historical figures. The mother of Mencius moved for several times to choose a good neighborhood for her son. Likewise, Mi's foster mother wept while taught him about the importance of a proper education. The formerly squandering Huangfu Mi was touched by his mother and finally became renowned writer, historian and medical specialist. As the old saying goes, "The determination to start fresh and redeem oneself is more valuable than gold."

【書淫】

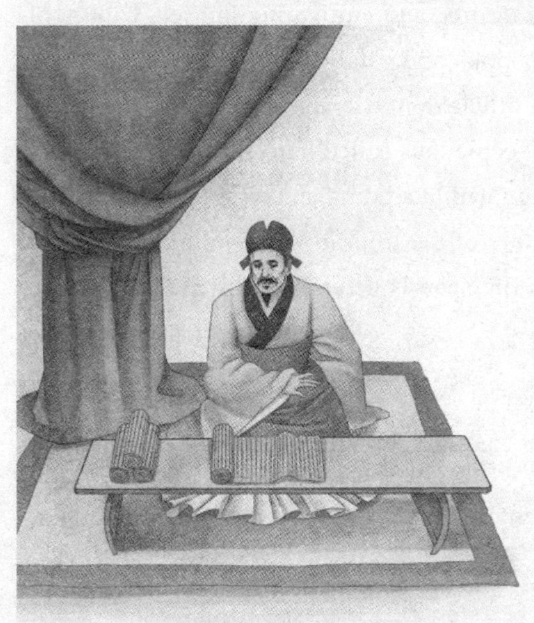

【原文】

（謐）沈①静寡欲，始有高尚之志②，以著述爲務，自號玄晏先生。……遂不仕。耽翫③典籍，忘寢與食，時人謂之"書淫"。或有箴④其過篤，將損耗精神，謐曰："朝聞道，夕死可矣⑤，况命之修短⑥分定⑦懸天乎！"

（選自《晉書·皇甫謐傳》）

【注釋】

①沈："沉"的異體字。②高尚之志：高潔自守、不願卑屈求仕的志向。此指著述之志。③耽翫：酷愛。翫，"玩"的異體字。喜愛。④箴（zhēn 針）：規勸。⑤"朝聞道"兩句：語出《論語·里仁》。⑥修短：長短。⑦分（fèn 奮）定：壽分確定。分，宿分，壽分。

【釋義】

皇甫謐性情沉静，少私寡欲，開始立下了高潔自守的志向，把著書立説當作己任，自己取號爲玄晏先生。……於是不出仕做官。他酷愛經典古籍，廢寢忘食，當時的人稱他爲"書淫"。有人規勸他過於愛讀書著述，將會損傷精神。皇甫謐説："早晨得知真理，就是晚間死去也滿足了，更何况壽命的長短定數是由上天决定呢？"

【按語】

大凡醫學名家，都是酷愛讀書的。張仲景"勤求古訓，博采衆方"，華佗"兼通數經"，孫思邈論《大醫習業》指出"凡欲爲大醫，又須涉獵群書"，李時珍"博學無所弗睍"等，無一例外。皇甫謐正是因爲立下了高潔自守、不願卑屈求仕的志向，决心一生以"著述爲務"，所以他才能酷愛典籍，廢寢忘食。無怪乎人們稱他爲"書淫"了。

【An Addict to Books】

Huangfu Mi was quiet, refrained from desires and cultivating himself with noble moral principles. Concentrated on writing books and establishing theories, he named himself Mr. Xuanyan and stayed away from officialdom. He was fond of the classics, so much as that he often forgot to eat or sleep. People thus called him an "addict to books" . Some people warned him that being too committed to reading and writing would exhaust him mentally. Huangfu Mi said, "If I were told of the truth in the morning, I would die happily in the evening. What's more, one's life span is determined by the god and one cannot do anything about it."

From *The Book of the Jin Dynasty* .

Editor's Note:

Most famous doctors and experts of any sort loved to read, such as Zhang Zhongjing, Hua Tuo, Sun Simiao and Li Shizhen. Huangfu Mi set high standards of researching, reading and writing for the later generations.

【不以酒肉爲禮】

【原文】

城陽①太守梁柳，謐從姑②子也，當之③官，人勸謐餞之④。謐曰："柳爲布衣時過⑤吾，吾送迎不出門，食不過鹽菜，貧者不以酒肉爲禮。今作郡而送之，是貴城陽太守而賤梁柳，豈中⑥古人之道？是非吾心所安也。"

（選自《晉書 · 皇甫謐傳》）

【注釋】

①城陽：郡名。故址在今山東莒縣。 ②從姑：父親的堂姊妹。 ③之：前往。 ④餞之：爲他餞行。餞，用酒食送行。 ⑤過：拜訪。 ⑥中（zhòng 衆）：符合。

【釋義】

被任命爲城陽太守的梁柳，是皇甫謐堂姑的兒子，要去赴任就職時，有人勸皇甫謐爲他餞行。皇甫謐說："梁柳做百姓時來拜訪我，我迎送他從不出門，飯食不外是鹹菜而已，清貧的人不把酒肉當作禮節。現在他做了郡守就爲他餞行，這是認爲城陽太守這個職務高貴而輕視了梁柳本人，難道符合古人做人的原則嗎？這是不讓我心安的事情。"

【按語】

在一般人看來，能爲做官的親友餞行或接風，是很愜意的事。因爲這是一種身份的顯示，故不少人樂此不疲。而在皇甫謐眼裏，"官帽"並不重要，他看重的是貧賤之交的親情。當年他的姑表兄弟梁柳爲布衣時，他"送迎不出門，食不過鹽菜"，而今梁柳升官做了城陽太守，他不願爲之餞行，仍然堅持"不以酒肉爲禮"。這才是古人所說的君子做人之道。

Wine and Meat do not Show the Courtesy

Liang Liu, the son of Huangfu Mi's aunt, was appointed the governor of Chengyang prefecture. When he was leaving for the position, some people advised Huangfu Mi to see him off. Huangfu Mi answered, "When Liang Liu visited me as a commoner, I never went out to meet or see him off and served him with only pickles. Poor people do not use wine and meat to show the courtesy. If I treat him differently now, I would be showing respect to his post, not to him as a person. Is this the moral principle of ancient sages? I would not feel at ease about that."

From *The Book of the Jin Dynasty* .

Editor's Note:

Common people would feel delighted to courteously see off or welcome their wealthy or important relatives. This way they felt important themselves. Not taking official ranks seriously, Huangfu Mi put more emphasis on the individuals themselves and family relations. He followed the doctrine of ancient sages by treating high officials equally with ordinary people.

【不封不樹】

【原文】

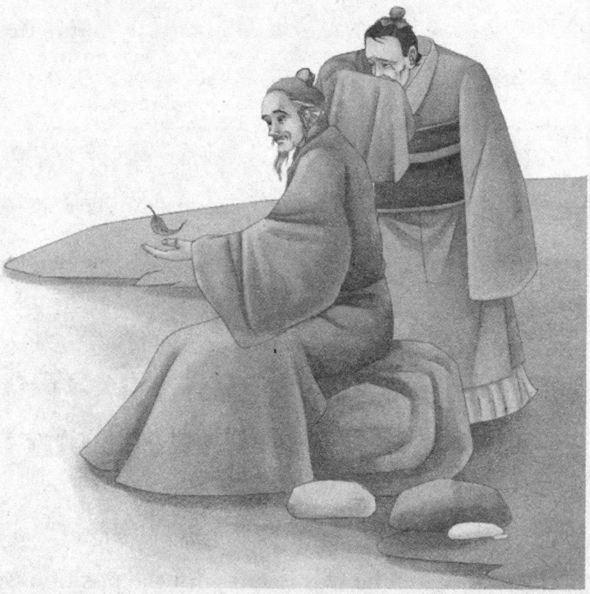

夫葬者，藏也①，藏也者，欲人之不得見也。而大爲棺槨②，備贈存物③，無異於埋金路隅而表於上也。雖甚愚之人，必將笑之。……《易》稱"古之葬者，衣之以薪④，葬之中野，不封不樹⑤。"是以死得歸真，亡不損生。故吾欲朝死夕葬，夕死朝葬，不設棺槨，不加纏斂⑥，不修⑦沐浴，不造新服，殯唅之物⑧，一皆絶之。吾本欲露形入坑，以身親土，或恐人情染俗來久⑨，頓革⑩理難。今故觕⑪爲之制。奢不石槨，儉不露形。……土與地平，還其故草，使生其上。無⑫種樹木、削除⑬，使生跡⑭無處，自求不知。……形骸與后土⑮同體，魂爽與元氣合靈，真篤愛⑯之至也。

（選自《晉書 · 皇甫謐傳》）

【注釋】

①藏也：《説文》，"葬，藏也。從死在茻中。"意思是葬就是埋葬屍體。以示意死在草叢中。②棺槨（guǒ 果）：内棺和外棺。槨，棺外的套棺。③備贈存物：把活着時的

物品大量用來陪葬。④衣之以薪：語出《周易·繫辭下》，一本作“厚衣之以薪”。意思是用柴草厚厚地覆蓋屍體。衣，覆蓋。活用作動詞。⑤不封不樹：不封土爲墳，不種樹以標其處。反映了上古時期薄葬的思想。⑥纏斂：纏裹屍身以入殮。斂,通“殮”。⑦修：建造。⑧殯唅（hàn 撼）：古代殯殮時，在死者口中放置珠玉。唅，通“琀”。含于死者口中的珠、玉之類。⑨或：又。染俗來久：受世俗影響由來已久。⑩頓革：立時改變。⑪觕：“粗”的異體字。⑫無：通“勿”。不要。⑬刪除：謂不要芟除墳上的雜草。⑭生跡：生前的痕跡。⑮后土：大地。⑯篤愛：厚愛。

【釋義】

皇甫謐在晚年一再强調，死後要節葬，反對厚葬。他說：葬，就是埋藏的意思，想讓人不能看見屍體。如果大造墳墓棺槨，詳備生前豪華之物以陪葬，這就等于把金銀埋在路邊而在地面標上字樣，引誘別人來盜取。即使非常愚蠢的人，也一定會恥笑他。……《周易》說：“古時埋葬死人，只用柴草覆蓋屍體，葬在荒野之中，不封土造墳，不種樹以標其處。”于是，死後能返璞歸真，性命亡了，不至于損傷身體。所以我想，如果早晨死，晚上就埋葬；如果晚上死，第二天早晨就埋葬。不設内棺外棺，對屍身不加纏裹而入殮，不興建沐浴之所，不縫製喪葬的服裝，殯殮時唅珠玉之事，一概摒絶。我本來想裸露形體入墓坑，用身體親近泥土，又恐怕人情受世俗影響由來已久，立時改變，情理難容。所以如今粗略地定個原則，奢侈不用套棺，儉約不露形體。……墓上的土要與地面持平，不要封土建墳，還原地面的青草，使它們生長在墓上。在墓上不要種植樹木，以作標記，不要芟除墓上的雜草，要使我生前的痕跡無處可尋，我自求人們不在意我，不必知道我埋葬的地方。讓我的形體與大地同體，讓我的魂靈與大自然的元氣融合在一起，這才真是對我的厚愛之至。

【按語】

在封建時代，統治者倡導厚葬。帝王將相，達官貴人，往往豪建墓地，大爲棺槨。上行下效，于是形成了一種奢靡的厚葬習俗。而著名的文學家和醫學家皇甫謐却拔出流俗，堅决反對厚葬，主張薄葬。他倡導上古聖人之風，“衣之以薪，葬之中野，不封不樹。是以死得歸真”。他認爲只有這樣，才能使形體與大地同體，靈魂與大自然的元氣融合在一起，此乃“真篤愛之至也”。這絶非簡單的節約葬禮，而蘊含着深厚的文化内涵。充分展示了這位大儒大醫博大的胸懷。今天，仍給我們有益的啓示。

No Tombs, No Trees

In his late years, Huangfu Mi repeatedly stressed that people should be buried simply instead of luxuriously after death. He argued as follows. To bury is to hide the deceased from the living and to bid eternal farewell. Decorating tombs and coffins elaborately with luxurious items inside is like burying gold by the roadside to invite theft. It does not take much intelligence to see the stupidity in this. "In antiquity," as argued in the *Book of Change*, "Dead bodies are covered by firewood only and laid in wasteland without tombs or trees marking their existence." This is for one to return to simplicity without causing extra trouble or cost for the living. Therefore, if I die in the morning, I would like to be buried in the evening; if I die in the evening, I would like to be buried by next morning. No layers of coffins, no covers on my body, and no precious item on my tongue are necessary. Nor do I wish to be bathed or finely clothed. Let nothing burden me. I would rather enter the tomb naked to get myself close to the soil, but this would not be accepted by the institutionalized social customs. Therefore, here is what I have planned for my deceased self: I do not need expensive stone coffins, as long as my body is hugged in the earth. Nor do I need elevated grave and trees, as long as what was originally growing in the soil returned, now with me in there. Let no one trim the grass, and let no one know where I am. I would like my body integrated into the earth, and my soul merged with the flowing energy of the nature. This way I would feel most deeply beloved and nurtured.

From *The Book of the Jin Dynasty* .

Editor's Note:

In ancient China, nobility and well-established individuals usually favored lavish funerals and thus led the trend of luxurious burials among ordinary people. However, Huangfu Mi, a highly regarded writer and medical expert, preferred a simple funeral. He thought that being buried in the wild could keep the body and soul integrated with the nature. The simple economical funeral conforms to the most profound aspects of Chinese culture, and demonstrates Huangfu's philosophical pursuits.

【醫道至重】

【原文】

夫受先人①之體，有八尺之軀，而不知醫事，此所謂游魂②耳！若不精通於醫道，雖有忠孝之心，仁慈之性，君父危困，赤子塗地③，無以濟之。此固聖賢所以精思極論④盡其理也。由此言之。焉可忽乎？

（選自晉·皇甫謐《針灸甲乙經》）

【注釋】

①先人：指亡故的父母。②游魂：漢魏之際的熟語，指苟延殘喘毫無定見之人。張仲景在《傷寒論序》中，曾指責那些不懂得醫道的人“遇災值禍，身居厄地，蒙蒙昧昧，蠢若游魂。”③赤子：本指初生嬰兒，此處泛指百姓。塗地：猶“塗炭”。塗，泥潭。喻遭受災難困苦。④精思極論：精密思考，透徹論述。

【釋義】

一個人稟受父母賜給的軀體，長着高大的個子，却不懂得醫學，這就是所說的沒有頭腦的人呀！假如對醫學道理不精通，即使有忠君孝親之心，有仁愛慈善的本性，當君主或父母病重，百姓遭災受難之時，也沒有辦法救助他們。這實在是聖賢們精密思考，透徹論述，詳盡探究醫學道理的原因。由此說來，怎麼可以忽視醫學呢？

【按語】

上自天子貴人，下至庶民百姓，誰能保證一生無恙？所以說醫道至重，它關係着天下民生。這也正是後人反復引用皇甫謐這段名言的原因。醫道是什麼？醫聖張仲景在《傷寒論序》中說：“上以療君親之疾，下以救貧賤之厄，中以保身長全，以養其生。”信然。

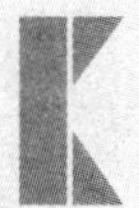

Medicine as the Supreme Doctrine

A person with a tall body granted by his parents would be soulless if not equipped with any basic medical understanding. If one is not versed in medical theory, even if he is loyal to the emperor and filial to his parents, kind-hearted and charitable, he could not save anyone when others suffer from illnesses. That was why the sages constructed sophisticated doctrines, had thorough discussions, and pursued the ultimate truth regarding the functioning of human body. Therefore, how can we ever ignore the study of medicine?

From *Canon of Acupuncture and Moxibustion*.

Editor's Note:

From nobility to ordinary people, no one can keep himself from suffering from diseases. Therefore, medical doctrines matter the most as they matter to human lives. People in later generations repeatedly quoted Huangfu Mi's words in this excerpt.

段醫簡封

【原文】

段醫[①]字元章，廣漢[②]新都人也。習《易經》，明風角。有一生來學積年，自謂略究要術，辭歸鄉里。醫爲合膏藥，並以簡書封於筒中，告生曰：“有急，發視之。”生到葭萌[③]，與吏争度。津吏撾[④]破從者頭。生開筒得書，言：“到葭萌，與吏鬥，頭破者，以此膏裹之。”生用其言，創者即愈。

（選自晉 · 干寶《搜神記 · 段醫》）

【注釋】

①段醫:《後漢書 · 段翳傳》等均作“段翳”,據 1979 年中華書局本《搜神記》改。

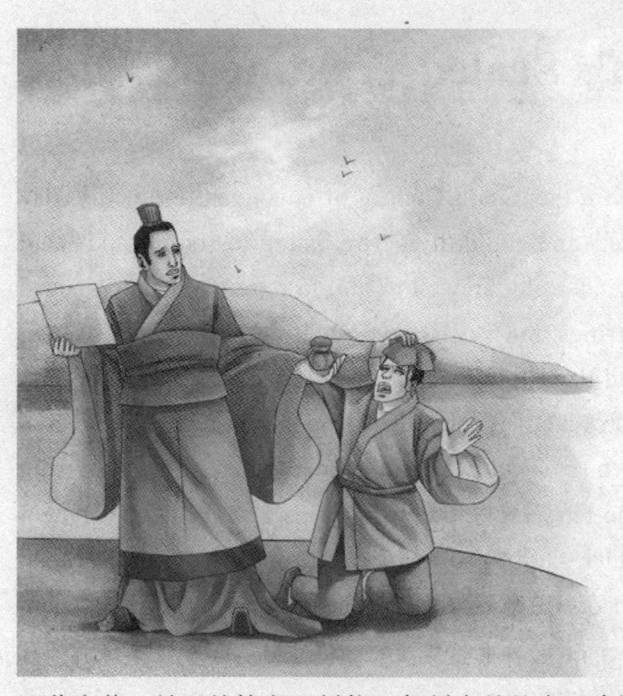

②廣漢：古廣漢郡，今屬四川廣漢。③葭（jiā 家）萌：廣漢郡有葭萌縣。④撾（zhuā 抓）：擊，打。

【釋義】

段醫，字元章，是廣漢郡新都縣（今四川省成都市新都區）人。他精通《易經》，懂得根據五音與四方之風聲來占吉凶的占候之術。有一個學生來學了好幾年，自以爲已經大致掌握了關鍵的道術，便辭別師傅回老家去。段醫給他配了些膏藥，並用竹簡寫了封信一起封在竹筒裏，告訴這學生説："碰上急事，就打開這竹筒看看。"這學生來到葭萌縣白水江邊，與官吏搶着渡河。管渡口的官吏打破了他隨從的頭。他打開竹筒看信劄，上面寫着："到葭萌縣，與官吏爭鬥，頭被打破的，就用這膏藥敷在傷口上。"他就按這話辦了，受傷的人馬上就痊愈了。

【按語】

東晉干寶（？—336）編撰的《搜神記》是中國古代志怪小説集。原本三十卷，已散佚，今存二十卷。所記多爲神靈怪異之事，也有一部分屬於民間傳説。故事大多篇幅短小，情節簡單，設想奇幻，極富浪漫主義色彩。干寶，字令升，新蔡（今屬河南）人。東晉史學家。

關於段醫簡封之事，《後漢書·段翳傳》也有類似記載，並説，那個學生對段醫更加嘆服，于是又返回學習，最終完成了學業。從中可以看出段醫的高超醫術，同时也告誡人們，學無止境，不要淺嘗輒止。清代名醫吳尚先在他的名著《理瀹駢文》中曾引用此典："寄諸遠道，偶同段翳之緘封。"意思是把它送給長途求醫的病人，作用也許與段翳封在竹筒裏的簡書相同。

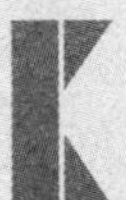

Doctor Duan's Sealed Treatment

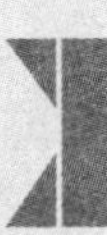

Doctor Duan Yuanzhang was from the Xindu County of Guanghan Prefecture. He had studied the *The Book of Change*[1] and could divine by listing to sounds and wind from four directions. One of his students bade farewell to him to return home, convinced that he had mastered the core doctrines and skills from Doctor Duan. Doctor Duan prepared some plasters for him, filled them in a bamboo tube together with a letter and told the student, "You can open the tube in emergency." The student passed by the Baishui River of Jiameng County and had a quarrel with a local official when he was crossing the river. The official in charge of the ferry broke the head of his attendant. The student opened the tube to read the letter, which said, "You will be confronted by a local official in Jiameng County. Apply the plaster on the person whose head is broken." The student acted accordingly and the wounded person soon recovered.

From *Anecdotes about Spirits and Immortals*.

Notes:

1. *The Book of Change* (《易經》/《周易》Yijing, aka Zhouyi): It is one of the most ancient Chinese classics. The book contains a divination system comparable to Western geomancy or the West African Ifá system, as well as a comprehensive set of philosophical values. Simplified versions of its division methods are still widely used in modern East Asia.

Editor's Note:

This excerpt was also recorded in the *Biography of Duan Yi* (《段翳傳》Duan Yi Zhuan) of *The book of the Later Han* (《後漢書》Houhanshu), which says that the student greatly admired Doctor Duan, and thus returned and continued to learn from him. The story speaks for doctor Duan's superb medical skills as well as divination skills.

【診脈驚帝】

【原文】

郭玉①者，廣漢雒②人也……和帝③時，爲太醫丞④，多有效應。帝奇之，仍⑤試令嬖臣⑥美手腕者，與女子雜處帷中⑦，使玉各診一手，問所疾苦。玉曰："左陽右陰，脈有男女，狀若異人⑧，臣疑其故⑨。"帝嘆息稱善⑩。

（選自南朝 · 范曄《後漢書》）

【注釋】

①郭玉：東漢時針灸家。廣漢（今四川廣漢市）人。師承涪翁、程高。曾提出爲富貴人治病有"四難"：貴人自作主張，不聽醫者的治療，這是第一難；保養身體不小心謹慎，這是第二難；筋骨脆弱，不能接受藥物治療，這是第三難；貪圖安逸，厭惡勞動，這是第四難。②雒（luò 洛）：東漢縣名，今四川廣漢北部。③和帝：劉肇，89—105 年在位。④太醫丞：太醫令的下屬官。⑤仍：因而，乃。⑥嬖（bì 避）臣：皇帝寵愛的近侍。⑦雜處帷中：指男女混雜置身於帷帳之中。古代禮俗。男醫生給貴族女子診脈，設一帷幕，讓病人從帷幕中伸手出來，醫生診其脈而不睹其面。⑧異人：指性別不同的人。⑨故：緣故。⑩嘆息：贊嘆。稱善：稱好。

【釋義】

郭玉是廣漢郡雒縣人……東漢和帝時，任太醫丞，治病多有療效。和帝感到他的醫術很神奇，就試着叫手腕長得美的後宮寵臣與宮女混雜置身在帷幕裏，讓郭玉分別診察寵臣和宮女各一隻手的脈象，問病人患病的情況。郭玉診脈後説："左手是陽性脈，右手是陰性脈，脈象有男有女，其形狀好像是性別不同的人。我懷疑其中的緣故。"和帝聽後感到驚訝，連聲贊嘆稱好。

【按語】

范曄（398—445），字蔚宗，南朝宋史學家，順陽（今河南淅川南）人。《後漢書》記事上起漢光武帝劉秀建武元年（25 年），下訖漢獻帝建安二十五年（220 年），囊括東漢一代一百九十六年的歷史。是"二十四史"中著名的前四史之一。

東漢名醫郭玉神奇的診脈技術，使皇帝感到驚訝，連聲"嘆息稱善"。這一故事曾在民間廣爲流傳。據説清代乾隆皇帝也曾用此法測試當時的名醫黄坤載，坤載以"龍得鳳脈"而驚走，其神妙脈法，深受乾隆的賞識。

Doctor Guo Yu Impressed the Emperor

Guo Yu was a native of Luo County of Guanghan Prefecture. During the reign of Emperor He of the Eastern Han Dynasty, he was nominated to Taiyicheng (the title of an imperial medical officer). Emperor had heard that Guo was an outstanding doctor, and planned to test his pulse-taking skill. He asked a eunuch with soft, beautiful hands and a female servant in the inner court to hide behind a heavy curtain and called Guo Yu to take each of their hands, respectively. The emperor then asked about the patient's condition. Guo took the pulse and said, "The left hand is of Yin pulse and the right one of Yang pulse. The pulse suggested both male and female features, and it seemed a person with both sexes in one body. I'm bewildered." Emperor He was extremely impressed and praised him highly.

From *The book of the Later Han.*

Editor's Note:

In this famous anecdote, Guo Yu's supreme pulse-taking skill greatly impressed the emperor. It is said that Emperor Qianlong in the Qing Dynasty used the same method to test the famous doctor Huang Kunzai. Doctor Huang was surprised by "female pulse of the emperor" . Doctor Huang also won the praise and appreciation of the Emperor Qianlong.

謐序三都

【原文】

左太冲作《三都賦》①初成,時人互有譏訾②,思意不愜。後示張公③,張曰:“此《二京》可三④。然君文未重於世,宜以經高名⑤之士。”思乃詢求於皇甫謐,謐見之嗟嘆,遂爲作敘。于是先相非貳⑥者,莫不斂袵⑦述焉。

(選自南朝 · 劉義慶《世説新語 · 文學第四》)

【注釋】

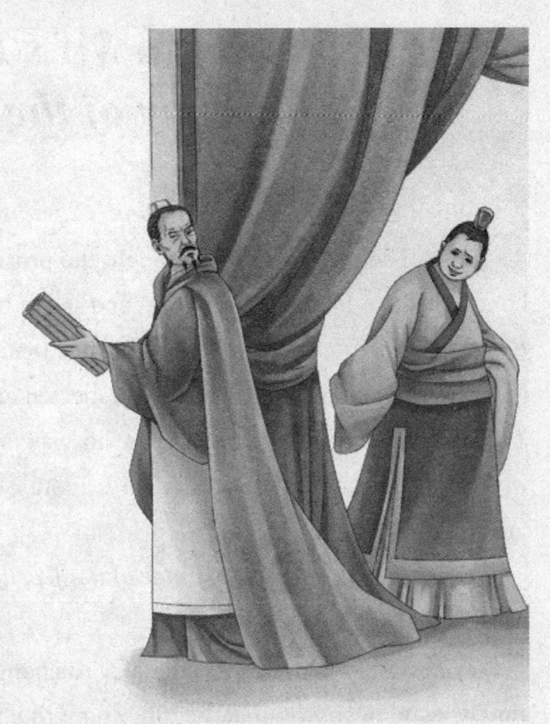

①太冲：左思的字。三都：指蜀都、吳都、魏都。②訾（zǐ 紫）：毀謗非議。③張公：即張華。西晉著名的學者，著有《博物志》十卷。④二京：指東漢張衡的《二京賦》。可三：可鼎足三立。⑤高名：指德高望重的名士。⑥非貳：非難懷疑。⑦斂衽（rèn 任）：整一整衣袖，表示尊敬。衽，衣襟。

【釋義】

左太冲（左思）剛寫成《三都賦》時，被當時的人交相嘲諷詆毀，左思心中不快。後拿給大學者張華看，張華說："這可以和張衡的《二京賦》鼎足而三了。然而你的文章還未被世人看重，應當有德高望重的名士提攜。"左思便去求教皇甫謐，皇甫謐看了《三都賦》後贊嘆不已，便爲之作敘。這樣一來，原來詆毀並懷疑他的人，無不恭敬地表示贊嘆。

【按語】

《世說新語》是由南朝宋劉義慶組織編寫的一部筆記小說。主要記敘了魏晉時代士大夫的言行及遺聞軼事，較多地反映了當時的思想、生活和清談放誕的風氣，對後世世說體作品的影響較大。該書所記個別事實雖不盡確切，但反映了門閥世族的思想風貌，保存了社會、政治、思想、文學、語言等多方面史料，價值很高。在中國文化史上佔有一定地位。

劉義慶(403—444)，南朝劉宋宗室，襲封臨川王，曾任荊州刺史、江州刺史等職。性好文，其他著述多種，均已散佚。

關於皇甫謐爲左思《三都賦》寫敘之事，在《晉書·皇甫謐傳》中早有記載，因謐作敘，左思的這篇傑作，很快流傳開來。"於是豪貴之家，競相傳寫，洛陽爲之紙貴。"成語"洛陽紙貴"即由此而來。由此可見，皇甫謐當時在文壇中的威望和影響。古人說：大醫者必大儒。從皇甫謐身上，再次印證了這一點。

Huangfu Mi's *Preface to the Rhapsody of the Three Capitals*

When Zuo Si[1] just wrote *Three Capitals' Rhapsody* , people of the time sneered at the prose. The dismayed Zuo brought the prose to a great scholar, Zhang Hua. Zhang told him, "This is a fine piece of work, and it can be compared to Zhang Heng[2]'s Rhapsodies *Eastern and Western Metropolis*. It is just that the common people have not seen the value in it yet. You should find a widely respected and famous person to introduce your work." Zuo Si then went to Huangfu Mi, who was amazed at the prose and wrote a preface for it. After that, people who had taken it lightly before all expressed their admiration of the prose.

From *A New Account of Tales of the World* [3].

Notes:

1. Zuo Si (左思 ca.250–305 aka Taichong): He was a writer and poet of the Western Jin Dynasty. In approximately 280, Zuo wrote the *Rhapsody of the Shu Capital* (《蜀都賦》 Shudu Fu), the first of his rhapsodies of capitals of the Three Kingdoms Period. People at the time admired this piece so much and hand-copied it so frequently that the price of paper in Luoyang was said to have risen as a result. This later gave rise to the Chinese idiom "Paper is Expensive in Luoyang" (洛陽紙貴), which was later used to praise a piece of literary work.

2. Zhang Heng (張衡 78–139) : He was an astronomer, mathematician, inventor, geographer, cartographer, artist, poet, and literary scholar from Nanyang of Henan Province. He lived during the Eastern Han Dynasty (東漢 25–220) of China. Zhang was one of the true polymaths in Chinese history, and in terms of prose alone, he was famous for the *Rhapsody of the Western Capital* (《西京賦》Xijing Fu), *Rhapsody of the Eastern Capital* (《東京賦》Dongjing Fu), and *On Returning to the Field* (《歸田賦》Guitian Fu), among others.

3. *A New Account of Tales of the World* (《世説新語》Shishuo Xinyu): It was compiled and edited by Liu Yiqing (劉義慶 403–444) during the Southern and Northern Dynasties (南北朝 420–589 A.D.) period. The book contains some 1,130 historical anecdotes and character sketches of some 600 literati, musicians, and painters who lived in the Han and Wei-Jin Periods, that is, the second through fourth centuries. It is both a biographical

source and a record of colloquial language of that time. The anecdotes and personalities are mostly attested in other sources. Traditional Chinese bibliographers, however, still treat this account as fiction for its informal style and sarcastic tone, rather than classify it as history.

Editor's Note:

This excerpt shows Huangfu Mi's prestige and influence in the literary world, in addition to being a distinguished doctor. It is said that great doctors had to be great scholars. Huangfu Mi was a perfect example.

【武后謝醫】

【原文】

唐高宗[①]苦風頭眩[②]，目不能視，召侍醫[③]秦鳴鶴診之，秦曰："風毒上攻，若刺頭出少血愈矣。"天后[④]自簾中怒曰："此可斬也！天子頭上豈是出血處耶？"鳴鶴叩頭請命。上曰："醫人議病，理不加罪。且我頭重悶，殆[⑤]不能忍，出血未必不佳。朕[⑥]意決矣。"命刺之。鳴鶴刺"百會"[⑦]及"腦户"[⑧]出血，上曰："我眼明矣。"言未畢，后自簾中頂禮[⑨]以謝之，曰："此天賜我師也！"躬負繒寶以遺之[⑩]。

（選自唐・胡璩《譚賓録》）

【注釋】

①唐高宗：即李世民之子李治，650—683年在位。②苦風頭眩：患頭眩暈。症見頭暈眼花，嘔逆發作無常，甚則厥逆。③侍醫：封建皇帝的保健醫生。即御醫。④天后：指武則天。⑤殆：幾乎。⑥朕（zhèn 振）：封建皇帝的自稱。⑦百會：穴名。在頭頂中央。⑧腦户：穴名。在枕骨上，强間後一寸五分處。⑨頂禮：以最尊敬的禮節表示謝意。⑩躬：親自。繒：古時對絲織品的總稱。遺（wèi 畏）：贈予，致送。

【釋義】

唐高宗得了眩暈病，頭暈目眩，不想睜眼，召太醫秦鳴鶴前來診治，秦鳴鶴診後說：

"風熱之毒上攻頭目，若用針點刺頭部少量出血即能痊愈。"皇后在簾内怒氣衝衝地說："你這個醫生該殺頭！皇帝的頭難道能放血嗎？"秦鳴鶴驚慌地磕頭請求饒命。皇上說："醫生議論病，按道理不應該治罪。況且我的頭目沉重煩悶，幾乎不能忍受，針刺頭上出血未必不好。我的主意已定。"便命令醫生扎針。鳴鶴針刺"百會"及"腦户"二穴出血。皇上說："我感覺眼睛清亮多了。"話還没有説完。皇后在簾内以最尊敬的禮節表示感謝説："這是老天爺恩賜的仙師呀！"説罷，親自背負精製的絲織品和珠寶，贈送給秦鳴鶴醫生。

【按語】

《譚賓録》十卷，本書多存唐一代朝野遺事，玄宗、肅宗、代宗、德宗四朝名臣軼事所記尤翔。多證實可信，有較高史料價值，新、舊《唐書》多有採録。撰者胡璩，字子温，唐代學者。爲唐文宗、武宗時人。

本文生動地記述了唐代御醫秦鳴鶴爲唐高宗治療眩暈病的故事。從中可以看出古代御醫的艱險生涯。雖然武后"頂禮以謝醫"，使秦鳴鶴受到恩賜，但已是死裏逃生，僥倖至此了。而武則天對御醫前後兩種截然不同的態度，充分顯示了她的機敏和狡詐。不免讓人發出"武后謝醫，心懷叵測"的感慨。

Empress Wu[1] Appreciated the Doctor's Work

Emperor Gaozong of Tang[2] had dizziness and had trouble opening his eyes. He summoned Doctor Qin Minghe to treat him. Qin Minghe examined him and said, "Wind and febrile toxins attacked your majesty's head and eyes. If I apply acupuncture on your head, and let some blood out, you will be cured." Empress said angrily behind the curtain, "you doctor should be killed! How dare you put needles into the emperor's head?" Qin Minghe kowtowed in panic and begged for mercy. The emperor said, "The doctor should not be punished since he was just trying to treat the disease. Moreover, my head and eyes feel unbearably heavy and burdened. Needling on the head to let it bleed a little may not be so bad. I've made up my mind." Then he asked the doctor to proceed. Minghe placed needles on the Baihui and Naohu points and let some blood out. The emperor said, "My eyes are clearer." Before he finished his words, Emperor Wu expressed her gratitude behind the curtain respectfully, saying, "What a talent blessed by the heaven!" Afterwards, she personally presented refined silk and jewelry to Doctor Qin Minghe.

From *A Collection of Anecdotes from the Tang Dynasty*.

Notes:

1. Empress Wu (武則天 Wu Zetian 624–705): She was the only female sovereign in Chinese history, who ruled under the name of her self-proclaimed "Zhou Dynasty" , from 690 to 705. Before that, she had served as the imperial concubine for Emperor Taizong of Tang and the Empress of Emperor Gaozong of Tang.

2. Emperor Gaozong of Tang (唐高宗 Tang Gaozong 628–683): He was the third emperor of the Tang Dynasty in China, ruling from 650 to 683 (although after January 665 much of the governance was in the hands of his second wife Empress Wu). Emperor Gaozong was the son of Emperor Taizong and Empress Zhangsun.

Editor's Note:

This excerpt recorded how the imperial doctor Qin Minghe treated the dizziness of Emperor Gaozong and reflects the precarious positions imperial doctors were in. Doctor Qin was fortunate as his treatment worked and the emperor trusted him. The polarized attitudes of the empress before and after the treatment demonstrated her caution and open-mindedness.

【劉張軼事】

【原文】

河間劉完素[①]病傷寒八日，頭痛脈緊，嘔逆不食，不知所爲。元素[②]往候，完素面壁不顧[③]。元素曰："何見待之卑[④]如此哉！"既爲診脈，謂之曰："脈病云云[⑤]。"曰："然"。"初服某藥用某味乎？"曰："然。"元素曰："子誤矣！某味性寒，下降走太陰，陽亡汗不能出。今脈如此，當服某藥則效矣。"完素大服，如其言遂愈。元素自此顯名。

（選自《金史 · 張元素傳》）

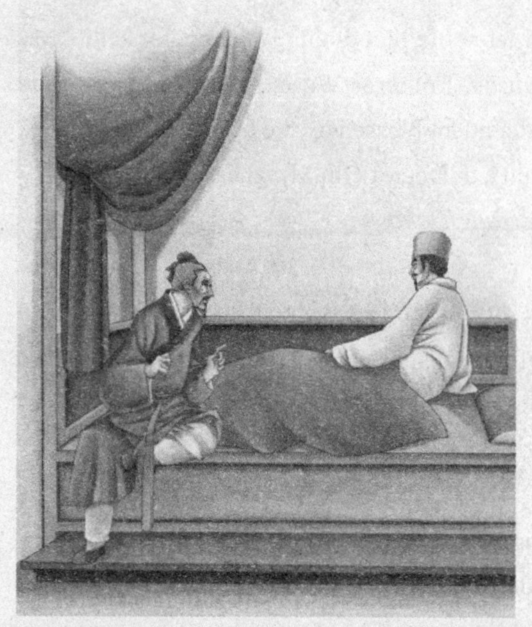

【注釋】

①河間：縣名，今河北省河間市。劉完素(约1120—1200)：字守真，號通玄處士，金元四大醫家之一。善用寒凉藥，以降心火益腎水爲主，稱寒凉派。著有《素問玄機原病式》《宣明論方》《傷寒直格》《傷寒標本心法類萃》《三消論》等。②元素：即張元素，字潔古，易州（今河北省易縣）人。金代著名醫家。其治學善化古方，自製新方，對藥性歸經、氣味、升降獨有創見。著有《醫學啓源》《臟腑標本藥式》《藥注難經》《珍珠囊》等。③面壁不顧：面朝着牆壁，不予理睬。④見待之卑：謂對客人瞧不起而不禮貌。⑤云云：猶言如此如此。

【釋義】

河間醫家劉完素患傷寒病已經八天了，仍然頭痛脈緊，嘔吐呃逆不願吃東西，自己不知怎樣治療才好。張元素聽説前去看望，劉完素面壁而卧，不予理睬。張元素説，“爲什麼這樣看不起人呢？”他爲劉完素診完脈，便把其脈象症狀如此如此説了一遍。完素説：“是這樣。”元素又接着説：“你以前一定是服了某某藥吧？”劉説：“是呀。”張元素説：“你錯了，某藥性寒，下降走太陰脾經，容易傷害脾氣，而陽氣衰微，汗不得出。現在脈象如此，應當服用某種藥物才能奏效啊。”劉完素被張元素這番話説得心服口服，就按張元素的意見服了藥，病就好了。從此以後，張元素的醫名就顯赫起來。

【按語】

《金史》是二十四史之一。撰成於元代，元代脱脱等主持編修。全書一百三十五卷，是反映女真族所建金朝的興衰始末的重要史籍。

以前人們常説：“同行是冤家”。金代醫家張元素，面對同行劉完素一時的傲慢，不計小節，以寬容的胸襟，抱着深厚的同道感情，爲完素治病。正是他的坦誠之心以及對病情的準確分析，打動了劉完素，才使劉順利地服其藥而把病治愈。最終“完素大服，元素自此顯名”，成就了杏林的一段佳話。

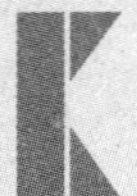

An Anecdote about Two Doctors

Liu Wansu, a physician in Hejian, suffered from typhoid fever for eight days. He had a headache, tight pulse, vomit, hiccups, and no appetite. He did not know how to treat himself. Hearing about his conditions, Doctor Zhang Yuansu went to visit him, but Liu Wansu stayed in bed, facing the wall and ignoring him. Zhang Yuansu said, "Why are you being so contempuous?" He felt Liu's pulse and speculated on Liu's symptoms. He was correct on all of them. Zhang then guessed what medicines Liu had been taking, and he was right on those as well. Zhang told Liu that he had been taking the wrong medicine, which was cold in nature, descending and harmful to the spleen, weakening the Yang Qi and restraining perspiration. He then suggested another type of medicine based on Liu's pulse. Impressed with Zhang, Liu Wansu took the medicine according to Zhang's prescription and then recovered. After that, Zhang Yuansu became famous in the medical field.

From *History of the Jin Dynasty*.

Editor's Note:

It was often said that people in the same occupation were rivals. Zhang Yuansu, did not mind the arrogance of his fellow physician, Liu Wansu, and treated his disease. His frankness and correct analysis of the disease touched and impressed Liu Wansu, who took Zhang's prescription and finally recovered. At last, Liu greatly admired Zhang, who won his reputation thereafter.

【東垣收徒】

【原文】

一日，謂友人周都運德父①曰："吾老，欲道傳後世，艱其人②奈何？"德父曰："廉台③羅天益謙父，性行敦樸，嘗恨④所業未精，有志於學，君欲傳道，斯人其⑤可也。"他日偕往拜之。君一見曰："汝來學覓錢醫人乎？學傳道醫人乎？"謙父曰："亦⑥傳道耳。"遂就學，日用飲食，仰給⑦於君。

（選自明 · 李濂《醫史 · 東垣老人傳》）

【注釋】

①德父：周都運的字。下文"謙父"是羅天益的字。②艱其人：難尋到合適的人。艱,難尋。用作動詞。③廉台：廉州。今河北省槁城。④嘗：通"常"。常常。恨：遺憾。⑤其：大概。⑥亦：只是。⑦仰給：依賴。

【釋義】

有一天，李東垣對友人周德父都運説："我年老了，想把醫術傳給後人，可是難尋到合適的人，怎麼辦呢？"德父説："廉州羅天益謙父，性情敦厚樸實，常常遺憾自己的醫道不精，有志學習，您想傳授醫道，這個人大概可以吧。"他日，周德父陪同羅天益一塊兒來拜見李東垣，李先生一見面就問："你是來學賺錢的醫生呢，還是學傳揚醫道的醫生呢？"羅天益回答："只是傳揚醫道罷了。"于是羅天益便得以跟從李東垣學醫，日用飲食，全依賴李先生供給。

【按語】

按常理説，醫生教學生，只要學生認真學習醫術，遵守規章制度，並按時交納學費就行了。至於學生將來想幹什麼，老師大可不去過問。而大醫李東垣則不然，他要求所收的弟子，必須有遠大的抱負，要做一個"傳道"的醫生，絶不收要做"覓錢醫生"的人爲弟子。這也正是他向友人周都運感嘆"欲道傳後世，艱其人奈何"的原因。而一旦選到合適的弟子，他不僅分文學費不收，而且對弟子的"日用飲食"全部承擔。從這裏，我們可以看到大師的博大情懷和崇高的境界。而今，東垣詢問弟子羅天益的話："汝來學覓錢醫人乎？學傳道醫人乎？"已經成了醫界名言。

Dongyuan Selecting a Disciple

After the war, Li Dongyuan returned to his hometown. One day, he told his friend Zhou Duyun, "I've become old. I would like to pass my medical skills to the later generation, but it is difficult to find a proper person. What should I do?" Zhou said, "Luo Tianyi, aka Qianfu, from Lianzhou, is honest and sincere. He often regrets about his insufficient medical training and is determined to further his study. If you want someone to pass on your medical knowledge, he's probably a suitable candidate." Later, Zhou accompanied Luo Tianyi to visit Li Dongyuan. Mr. Li asked Luo immediately after meeting them if he wanted to be a doctor for money or for inheriting the way of medicine. Luo Tianyi picked the latter. Li thus accepted Luo as his disciple, and provided him lodging and daily necessities.

From *A History of Chinese Medicine*.

Editor's Note:

Usually teachers expected students to learn earnestly, obey the rules and hand in tuitions in time, and paid little attention to students' future ambition. Doctor Li Dongyuan was different. He wanted his student to hold high ideals when pursuing medical studies, instead of seeking for money. This in turn showed the noble mind of Doctor Li himself as a medical specialist. His question for Luo became well-known in the medical circle and was later quoted by many people.

【朱謙葛雄】

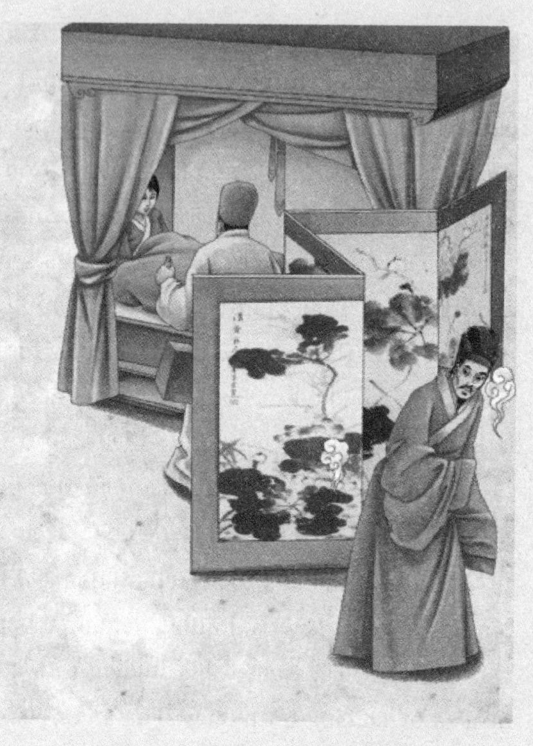

【原文】

朱彦修曾治浙中一女子病瘵[1]，且愈，頰上兩丹點不滅。彦修技窮，謂主人曰："須吳中葛公[2]耳。然其人雄邁不羈[3]，非子所致也。吾遣書往彼必來。"主人悦，具供帳舟楫[4]以迎。

使至，葛公方與衆博[5]大叫，使者侍立中庭。葛公瞪目視之曰："爾何爲者？"使者奉牘跪上[6]之，葛公省書，不謝客行，亦不返舍，遂登舟。

比至，彦修語其故，出女子視之。可久曰："法可刺兩乳。"主人難之。可久曰："請覆以衣。"援針[7]刺之，應手而滅。主人贈遺[8]甚豐。可久笑曰："吾爲朱先生來，豈責[9]爾報耶？"悉置不受。

（選自明 · 徐禎卿《異林》）

【注釋】

①朱彦修(1281—1358)：名震亨，婺州（今屬浙江）人。家居丹溪，人称"丹溪翁"。元代醫學家。瘵(zhài 寨)：痨病。②吳中：蘇州的别稱。葛公，指葛可久。葛乾孫(1305—1353)，字可久。元代著名醫家。③雄邁不羈：性情豪放，不受拘束。④具：置備。供帳舟：備有幔帳的小船。楫：划船的槳。⑤衆博：衆人賭博。⑥奉牘跪上：跪地捧信遞上。⑦援針：拿起針。⑧遺（wèi 畏）：贈予。⑨責：責求。

【釋義】

朱彦修曾給浙江中部的一位女子治療痨病，痨病將愈，只是面頰有兩個紅暈點不去。彦修用盡辦法，仍未去除。便對病家説："必須邀請蘇州葛可久先生才能治療。但是葛先生的性格豪放不受拘束，你是請不來的，我寫封信你們帶去，他必然前來診治。”病家甚喜，于是劃着備有幔帳的小船，前往迎請。

送信的人到了蘇州，看見葛可久先生正和多人賭博，大叫大嚷，便站在院中恭候。葛先生瞪眼看着來人說：“你是幹什麼的？”來人急忙兩膝跪地，捧信遞上，葛先生看完書信，没有告辭衆客，也没顧得回屋，就立即乘船前往。

等到葛可久來到病家，彦修立即介紹了治療情況，並唤出病人，讓葛先生診視。葛可久診後說：“按法，應當針刺兩乳。”病家聽了，感到爲難。葛先生說：“請給病人穿上一層衣服。”于是拿起針來，按穴刺入，病人兩頰紅暈點立即消失。病家贈送很多禮物表示感激。葛先生笑着說：“我是爲朱彦修先生來的，難道還責求你酬報嗎？”全部禮物放置原處，概不接受。

【按語】

徐禎卿（1479—1511），字昌穀，一字昌國，祖籍常熟梅李鎮，後遷居吳縣（今江蘇蘇州）。明代文學家，被人稱爲“吳中詩冠”，與祝允明、唐寅、文征明齊名，號稱“吳中四才子（亦稱江南四大才子）”。其詩格調高雅，有名句“文章江左家家玉，煙月揚州樹樹花”而爲人稱譽。徐禎卿後期信仰道教，研習養生。惜英年早逝，年僅33歲。著有《異林》《談藝録》《迪功集》等。

衆所周知，朱彦修爲金元四大家之一。據元代戴良《丹溪翁傳》記載：朱彦修曾跟隨大理學家朱熹的四傳弟子許文懿，學習道德性命學説，深受薰陶。他醫德高尚，“執心以正，立身以誠”，性情静謐，謙虚謹慎，善取他人之長。而葛可久出自中醫世家，藝精技絶，性格豪放，雄邁不羈，治病輒有奇效。他與朋友交而重道義，爲救病人而不計名利。朱氏謙謹，葛氏雄邁，二人的不同性格交相輝映，在本文中得到了形象的展示。而朱葛之間的深情厚誼，更令人欽敬。

二人相互切磋，相互督促，互相敬重，已在醫界傳爲佳話。

The Modest Zhu and the Heroic Ge

Zhu Yanxiu once treated a girl from Zhejiang who had tuberculosis. After she recovered from the disease, there were two red spots on her cheek. Zhu tried every method but could not have them removed. He told the family of the patient to send for Doctor Ge Kejiu from Suzhou. As Ge had a reputation of being bold and unconstrained, Liu wrote a personal letter to him and asked the girl's family to bring it to Ge. The patient's family members were greatly reassured, and went to invite Ge with nicely decorated boat.

The messenger arrived at Suzhou and found Mr. Ge gambling with many people and shouting. He thus waited respectfully in the yard. Mr. Ge glared at the messenger and asked, "What are you doing here?" The messenger hastily kneeled down to present the letter. After reading the letter, without bidding farewell to the guests, without returning to the room to prepare, Ge immediately boarded the boat and came to the patient's residence.

Upon Ge's arrival, Zhu immediately introduced to him the situation and called out the patient for treatment. Mr Ge examined her and said, "Her breasts should be needled for treatment." The patient's family members felt embarrassed. Mr. Ge said, "Put a layer of clothes on the patient." He then proceeded with the treatment, and the red spots soon disappeared. The patient's family presented many gifts to express their gratitude. Mr. Ge laughed and said, "I came here upon Zhu Yanxiu's request, not for your reward." He refused to take any gift.

From *Records of Extraordinary Things*.

Editor's Note:

As one of the greatest figures during the Jin and Yuan Dynasties, Zhu Yanxiu once learned morality and medicine from Xu Wenyi, the fourth generation student of the great scholar and philosopher, Zhu Xi. With noble mind, calm personality, modesty and caution, Zhu was good at learning from others' strengths. By contrast, Ge Kejiu, the descendant of a medical family, had proficient skills and bold personality. He valued morality and justice instead of fame and money. This excerpt vividly portrayed both Doctor Zhu's modesty and Doctor Ge's boldness. People in the medical circle greatly admire their friendship and mutual respect.

【東垣附柬】

【原文】

湖南士人以謁選過泗州[①]，有通《太素脈》[②]者診之，云："公將來得官，然有病不治。"士竦[③]然曰："何病？"曰："病疽[④]。"士求示藥方。脈者翻覆群書，凝思晝夜，竟不得其法。留五日別去，脈者送之曰："到京訪東垣[⑤]或有生理。"明年，士果得第[⑥]，即謁東垣，時東垣尚未知名，才按指，駭曰："公脈哮數[⑦]，毒氣中藏，將不食新[⑧]矣！"士具告以泗州之語，東垣笑曰："渠[⑨]知我，且以相試也。"亦停思數刻，謂士人："此時梨正熟，君能噉[⑩]幾許？速買，率意噉之，旬日後報我。"士如言恣噉，復往謁東垣，望見即言："病已減半矣。"因問："噉幾何？"曰："二百。"曰："尚未。"更旬日，東垣喜曰："今幸無恙，但發瘡耳。"未三日，遍體生疥，亦尋[⑪]愈，遂出都門[⑫]。東垣附柬[⑬]報泗州，泗州北向拜曰："非吾所及，莫謂天下無人也。"

（選自明 · 徐樹丕《識小録》）

【注釋】

①謁選：赴京進見，等待選拔。謁，進見。泗州：今江蘇東北部和安徽北部一帶，相當於宿遷、泗陽、泗縣等地。②《太素脈》：診脈專書。③竦：通"悚"。恐懼。④疽：癰瘡。⑤東垣：即李杲（1180—1251），字明之，自號東垣老人。真定（今河北正定縣）人，金元四大家之一。從師張元素，創内傷學説，譽爲"補土派"。著有《脾胃論》《内外傷辨惑論》《蘭室秘藏》等。⑥得第：科舉考中。⑦脈哮數：脈象促躍而速。⑧不食新：吃不上新糧食了。⑨渠：他，彼。⑩噉(dàn 淡)：同"啖"。吃。⑪尋：很快。⑫都門：京都的城門。此指北京。⑬柬：書信。

【釋義】

湖南的一位讀書人，進京待選路過泗州，有位精通《太素脈》的人爲他診斷説："先生將有官運，但得病不易治療。"讀書人恐懼地問道："要得什麼病啊？"診者説："要患癰疽。"讀書人請求藥方，診者查閲了很多醫書，又聚精會神地考慮了一天一夜，最終也没想出治法來。讀書人等了五天，辭别而去。診者送行時對讀書人説："先生到了京城，可拜訪李東垣，他或許能給您治好。"第二年，讀書人果然科舉考試得中，就去拜訪李東垣，當時李東垣尚無醫名，剛一診脈，便驚訝地說：“你的脈促躍而急，毒氣侵於内臟，恐怕吃不上新糧食了！”這位讀書人便把泗州之事告訴了李東垣，東垣笑着說：“他怎麼了解我呢？暫且試治一下吧。”于是考慮了好久，告訴讀書人説：“現在梨正熟，快去買來，儘量吃，十天後再來告訴我。”讀書人遵着東垣的話儘量吃梨，過了十天又去拜訪東垣，東垣一見面就說：“病情好了一半。”又問：“吃了多少梨呀？”讀書人說：“二百個。”東垣說：“病還没痊愈。”又過了十天，東垣高興地說：“今幸而無大礙，只是會出現瘡疹罷了。”没過三天，讀書人全身生疥，很快就好了。讀書人離開京城回家，李東垣順便寫了一封書信交給他，讓他路過泗州時送交予精《太素脈》的人。精《太素脈》者收悉信後，便面向北方拱手作揖說：“東垣先生的醫術，我是不能比擬的，不要説天下没有能人呀！”

【按語】

《識小録》爲明清之際徐樹丕著的筆記。徐樹丕，明末學者，號活埋庵道人。生平不詳。

本文通過治愈湖南士人癰疽病的事例，表現了李東垣的精妙醫術和泗州醫生推薦賢能的美德。泗州醫生誠心推薦東垣，東垣附柬又謝意泗州，全是爲病人着想。這充分展現了我中華民族文明謙讓的禮儀風范。值得一提的是，本文爲我們提供一例啖梨愈風的病例。宋代孫光憲所著《北夢瑣言》卷十也講述了“啖梨愈風”的病例。

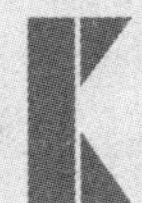

A Letter from Doctor Li Dongyuan

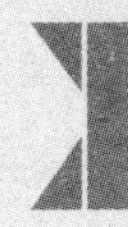

A scholar in Hunan went to the capital for the imperial examination. When he passed Sizhou, a person with a good command of *The Taisu Pulse* [1] diagnosed him, saying, “You are going to be an official, but you will suffer from a disease that is difficult to treat.” The scholar asked with fear, “What kind of disease?” The man answered, “A terrible carbuncle.” The scholar asked for medication. The man referred to many medical books and pondered on possible treatments for a day and a night, but could not find one that would work. The scholar waited for five days before resuming his journey. The man said to the scholar when seeing him off, "You could visit Li Dongyuan in the capital. He might be able to cure your disease." The next year, the scholar passed the imperial examination indeed, and he visited Li Dongyuan, who was not yet famous. Li felt his pulse and said in astonishment, "Your pulse is rapid and bouncing, indicating the attack of toxic Qi in the viscera. You might not be able to eat the grains of next harvest season." The scholar told Li about the diagnosis he had received and the mysterious man in Sizhou. Li laughed and answered, "How did he know about me? I'll give it a try then."

Li thought for quite a while and told the scholar, "Pears are ripe at present. Buy some and eat as much as possible, and then come to see me in ten days." The scholar followed Dongyuan's words and came back after ten days. Upon meeting him, Dongyuan said, "Half way there in having you cured." Then he asked, "How many pears have your eaten?" The scholar answered, "Two hundred." Dongyuan said, "Continue with the treatment." After another ten days, Dongyuan met him and said delightedly, "Fortunately there will not be any big problem, though you will develop scabies." Three days later, the scholar had scabies all over his body but soon recovered. When the scholar left the capital for home, Li Dongyuan asked him to deliver a letter to the man with a good command of *The Taisu Pulse* in Sizhou. After reading the letter, the man bowed facing the north and said, "I feel so humbled by the medical skill of Doctor Li Dongyuan. Who says there is no talent in this world?"

From *Records of Trivial Affairs* .

Notes:

1. *The Taisu Pulse* (《太素脈》 Taisu Mai) : A book written by Zhang Taisu in the Ming Dynasty, which was a systematic work about the function and treatments pertaining to the Taisu pulse. It was said that Taisu pulse has connection with people's fates and fortunes.

Editor's Note:

This excerpt demonstrates the outstanding medical skills of Li Dongyuan, and praises the Sizhou doctor's virtue of recognizing and recommending great talents. We can speculate that Li Dongyuan's letter contained a message of gratitude and the method of curing carbuncles with pears.

【桐葉催生】

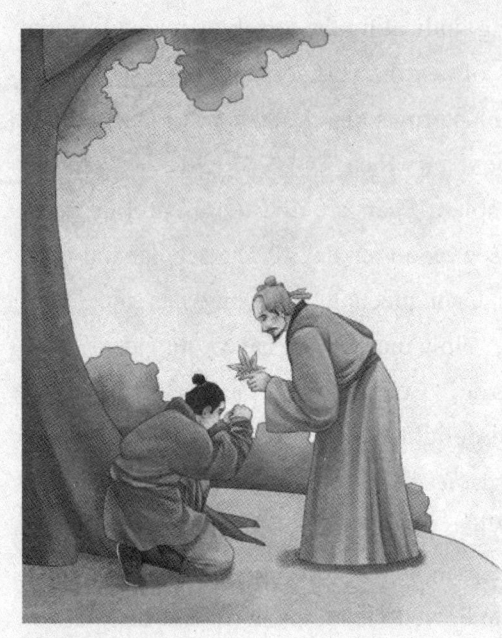

【原文】

滑壽[①]字伯仁，號櫻寧，工古文詞，善醫。……其治人疾，不拘于方書，而以意處劑，投無不立效。秋日，姑蘇[②]諸仕人[③]邀游虎丘山[④]。一富家有產難，挽回[⑤]，諸仕人不可。先生登階[⑥]，見新落梧桐葉，拾與之曰："歸急以水煎而飲之。"未登席[⑦]，報兒產矣。皆問此出何方，櫻寧曰："醫者意也，何方之有？夫妊已十月而未產者，氣不足也。桐葉得秋氣而墜，用以助之，其氣足，寧[⑧]不產乎？"

（選自明・許浩《復齋日記》）

【注釋】

①滑壽：元末明初醫学家，祖籍襄城（今屬河南）人。後遷儀真（今江蘇儀征）和余姚（今浙江）。有《讀素問鈔》《難經本義》《診家樞要》《十四經發揮》等著作傳世。②姑蘇：今蘇州市。因蘇州西南有姑蘇山而得名。③仕人：做官的人。④虎丘山：在蘇州市西北。相傳吳王闔閭葬於此。有虎丘塔、雲岩寺、劍池、千人石等古跡。⑤挽回：拉他回去。⑥階：石臺階。⑦未登席：尚未就座宴飲。⑧寧：怎麼，難道。

【釋義】

滑壽，字伯仁，號櫻寧生，自幼靈敏好學，攻習文詞，後精醫學。……他給人治病，不拘泥古方書，而是根據病情靈活立方，用藥無不顯效。有一年秋天，蘇州一些做官的人，邀請滑壽先生同游虎丘山。有一富家孕婦難産，想拉他回家診治，同游的人們不讓他走。這時滑先生走到石臺階上，正當一片梧桐葉落地，于是他拾起來交給病家說："拿回去趕快用水煎梧桐葉做湯喝下。"游山的人們還沒有坐下宴飲，病家就回來說小兒已生下來。同游的人都驚奇地詢問滑壽此方出於何書，滑壽說："醫就是'意'的意思，以意度之，哪有一定之方啊。凡婦女懷孕，超過十個月臨産，是氣虛的緣故。梧桐葉得金秋肅降之氣而落，煎湯借其肅降之氣以輔助産婦之正氣，産婦正氣足了，哪有不順利生産的道理呢？”

【按語】

《復齋日記》二卷，記敘明初以來朝野事迹的筆記。明代許浩撰，其生平不詳。

秋氣肅降，萬物凋零。滑壽借用梧桐葉得金秋肅降之氣而催産。其用之妙，讓人嘆服。而後人用梧桐葉催産而不效者，是因爲脱離了特定的時間和環境，即“非其時也”。

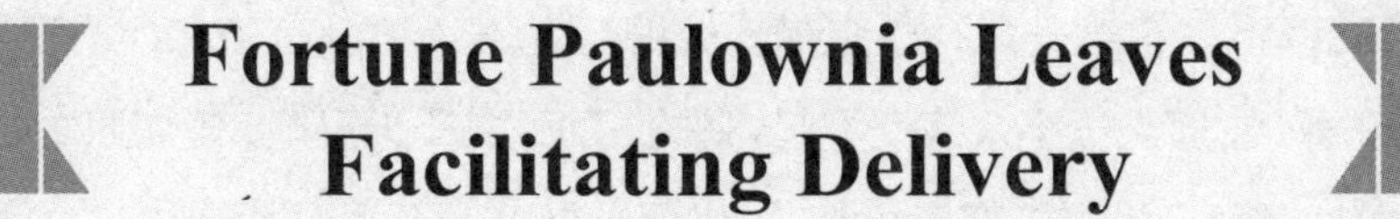

Fortune Paulownia Leaves Facilitating Delivery

Hua Shou, aka Boren or Yingningsheng, was keen and diligent in learning, first specialized in literature and then proficient in medicine. He treated people with flexibility based on the patients' specific conditions, not constrained by established rules or written medical formula. One day, some officials in Suzhou invited Doctor Hua Shou to visit the Huqiu Mountain. A pregnant woman from a wealthy family had severe trouble in labor, and sent someone for Hua. Hua's official friends would not let him leave. Doctor Hua stepped onto a stone stair, when a leaf fell on the ground from a Paulownia fortunei Hemsl. Hua picked it up, handed it to the messenger and said, "Take these leaves home and decoct them with water, then have the patient taken the decoction." Before Hua and his company had dinner, the messenger came back with the good news that a baby had been born. Everyone was impressed and asked Hua what formula he gave to the woman. Doctor Hua answered, "The word for medicine sounds like the word for meaning for a reason. I just did some speculation, and did not prescribe any formula. Pregnant women with Qi deficiency would deliver after ten months. The Fortune Paulownia leaves fall because of the descending Qi of the autumn. The descending Qi could facilitate the delivery process. And that's why the leaves treatment worked."

From *Diaries of Fuzhai*.

Editor's Note:

Hua got the inspiration from the falling Fortune Paulownia leaves and came up with a miraculous treatment. People of later generations used the same method but failed because they did not keep in mind the particular time and environment that made this treatment work.

【薛雪妙術】

【原文】

吳門名醫薛雪[①]，自號一瓢，性孤傲，公卿延之不肯往，而予有疾，則不招自至。乙亥[②]春，余在蘇州，庖人王小余病疫不起，將掩棺而君來，天已晚，燒燭照之，笑曰："死矣！然吾好與疫鬼戰，恐得勝亦未可知。"出藥一丸，搗石菖蒲汁調和，命輿夫有力者用鐵箸[③]鍥其齒灌之。小餘目閉氣絶，喉汩汩然[④]似咽似吐。薛囑曰："好遣人視之，鷄鳴時當有聲。"已而果然。再服二劑，而病起。

乙酉冬，余又往蘇州，有厨人張慶者，得狂易之疾，認日光爲雪，啖少許，腸痛欲裂，諸醫不效。薛至，袖手向張臉上下視曰："此冷痧也，一刮而愈，不必診脈。"如其言，身現黑瘢如掌大，亦即霍然[⑤]。余奇賞[⑥]之。先生曰："我之醫即君之詩，純以神行[⑦]，所謂人居屋中，我來天外是也。"

（選自清 · 袁枚《隨園詩話》卷五）

【注釋】

①薛雪：字生白，號一瓢，清代著名的醫學家，與袁枚交往甚深。②乙亥：1755年。③輿夫：轎夫。箸：筷子。④汩汩然：水響聲。⑤霍然：消散的樣子。多用以形容病愈之速。⑥賞：稱賛。⑦神行：精神運作。此謂運用自如。

【釋義】

吳縣（今江蘇省蘇州市郊）城裏的名醫薛雪，自號一瓢。個性孤僻高傲，三公九卿等大官請他都不肯前往；但是我有病，却不用招請他自動會來。乙亥年春天，我在蘇州。厨師王小余患疫病一病不起，快要閉棺時他到來。當時天色已晚，他點燃蠟燭照看王小余，笑着說："死啦！但是我喜歡跟疫鬼作戰，說不定可以取得勝利。"遂拿出一丸藥，搗石菖蒲汁來調和，叫有力氣的車夫，用鐵筷撬開他的牙齒灌藥。王小余雙目緊閉氣已斷絶，喉嚨中汩汩地好像咽又好像吐。薛雪囑咐說："好生派人看護他，鷄叫天亮時應當會有聲息。”不久果真如此。又服兩劑藥，病就痊愈。

乙酉年冬天，我又到蘇州。有個叫張慶的厨師，得了精神病，誤認日光是雪，吃一點點東西，腸子痛得像裂開來一樣。衆醫治療無效。薛雪趕到，袖着手上下觀察張慶説："這是冷痧，刮一刮就會好，用不着切脈。"按照他的話刮痧，身上刮出像手掌般大的黑斑，病也就很快好了。我非常贊賞他的醫術。先生説："我治病，好比你寫詩，純熟到家後就能運用自如。所説的'人居屋中，我來天外'就是這個意思。"

【按語】

袁枚（1716—1798）：字子才，號簡齋，世稱隨園先生，錢塘（今浙江杭州）人。清代著名文學家，乾隆進士。三十三歲辭官并退居於南京附近的小倉山自建的隨園，直至逝世。著有《小倉山房集》《隨園詩話》等。

本文通過袁枚親見的兩則病例，表現了清代大醫薛雪爐火純青的高妙醫術和圓通睿智、詼諧幽默的性格。從中我們可以深切地感受到，清代文學家袁枚與醫學大師薛雪兩位朋友之間的深情厚誼，同時也能體會到，醫學和文學的異曲同工之妙。

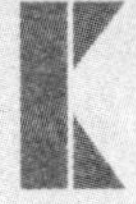

Xue Xue's Magical Cure

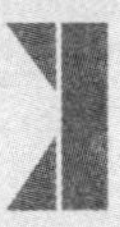

The famous doctor Xue Xue from Wu County, who called himself Yipiao, was eccentric and arrogant. Even high-ranking officials could not get a visit with him, but whenever I am in need, he would come without invitation. One spring, I was in Suzhou. My cook Wang Xiaoyu suffered from an epidemic disease and soon died. When people were ready to close his coffin, Xue Xue came at night, examined Wang with candles, laughed and said, "He is dead! But I like to fight with the ghost of epidemic, and maybe I'll win." He then brought out a pill, combined it with grassleaf sweetflag rhizome (*Rhizoma Acori Tatarinowii*) juice, and asked a strong wheeler to unclench Wang's teeth with iron chopsticks and poured the medicine in. With his eyes tightly closed and breath stopped, Wang Xiaoyu seemed to be swallowing or vomiting, judging from the sound in his throat. Xue Xue said, "Find someone to take care of him. He'll regain consciousness at dawn." He was right. After taking another two doses of medicine, Wang recovered.

In one winter, I came to Suzhou. Another cook named Zhang Qing suffered from a mental illness. He would mistake the sun as the snow and had a bursting pain in his intestines. No doctor could cure him until Xue Xue came. He casually examined Zhang Qing and said, "This is cold cholera. Pulse taking is not necessary. Just scrape his skin to extract the toxins." Thanks to his suggestions, the patient recovered soon with palm-large spots on the body left from the scraping. I admired his medical expertise very much. Xue said, "I treat diseases just like you write poems. It was mind at work after enough training and practice. That is what people mean when they say 'Masters achieve amazing results faraway even when they are physically confined in one room'."

From *Yuan Mei's Comments of Poetry* .

Editor's Note:

The excerpt is written by Yuan Mei, a great master of literature from the Qing Dynasty, and records his personal experiences with the outstanding doctor Xue Xue (薛雪 1681-1770). These stories also speak for Yuan and Xue's friendship and mutual trust.

【葉薛結怨】

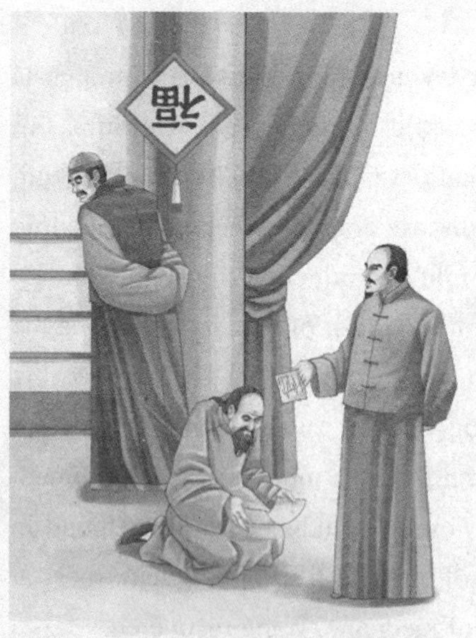

【原文】

乾隆[1]間，吳門[2]大疫，郡[3]設醫局以濟貧者，諸名醫日一造[4]也。有更夫[5]某者，身面浮腫，遍體作黄白色，詣[6]局求治。薛生白[7]先至，診其脈，揮[8]之去，曰："水腫已劇，不治。"病者出，而葉天士[9]至，從肩輿[10]中遙視之，曰："爾非更夫耶？此爇[11]驅蚊帶受毒所致，二劑可已[12]。"遂處方與之。薛爲之失色[13]。因有"掃葉莊""踏雪齋"之舉。二人以盛名相軋[14]蓋由於此。

（選自陸以湉《冷廬醫話》）

【注釋】

①乾隆：清高宗弘曆的年號，1736—1795年在位。②吴門：舊時蘇州的别稱。③郡：城。地方行政區域。④日一造：每天去一次。⑤更夫：舊時負責打更的人。⑥詣：到。⑦薛生白：名雪，號一瓢，清代著名醫學家，江蘇吴縣（今蘇州）人，與葉天士齊名。⑧揮：擺手。⑨葉天士：名桂，號香岩，江蘇吴縣（今蘇州）人，清代著名醫學家。⑩肩輿：兩人抬的轎子，形同圈椅。⑪爇（ruò若）：點燃。⑫已：痊愈。⑬失色：變了臉色。⑭相軋：互相排擠。

【釋義】

清朝乾隆年間，蘇州一帶疫病大流行，當地政府設置醫局以免費救治貧苦百姓，當地名醫都每天必去應診一次。有一打更的人，身面浮腫，渾身發黄，前來醫局求醫。薛生白先生先診其脈，斷爲不治之症，擺了擺手説："你這水腫病已經很重了，不好治了。"更夫出門，正巧碰上葉天士來到，天士在轎中遠遠看見便問道："你不是那位打更的人嗎？你這病是燃燒柴薪熏蚊時受毒所致，服兩劑藥就會好的。"説罷立即給他開了藥方。薛生白見此情景，大爲失色。後來因嫉妒葉天士，把書房改爲"掃葉莊"三字。葉天士聽説後，就把自己的書房改名"踏雪齋"。葉、薛二人都是名醫，而互相排擠，乃始於此。

【按語】

陸以湉，清代桐鄉（今浙江嘉興）人，晚清著名醫家。所著《冷廬醫話》，成書於1858年，全書分五卷。陸氏所載醫史文獻資料豐富，論述精廣，並多個人識見，故在醫話著作中素負盛譽。

葉桂和薛雪結怨，及"掃葉莊""踏雪齋"之舉，是否確有其事，也可能是人云亦云之訛傳，姑且不去考究。這個故事本身則給人以深刻的啓示。三國時曹丕在《典論·論文》中説過一段意味深長的話："文人相輕，自古而然。……是以各以所長，相輕所短。里語曰：'家有弊帚，享之千金'。斯不自見之患也。"所謂"不自見"，就是不能正確對待自己。那麼，怎樣才能避免這種毛病呢？曹丕又説"蓋君子審己以度人，故能免於斯累。"此語發人深思。只有"審己以度人"，才能正視自己的短處，發現别人的長處。醫生之間，不也是同樣道理嗎？

A Feud between Two Doctors

During the reign of Emperor Qianlong in the Qing Dynasty, an epidemic disease spread in the Suzhou area. The local government set up temporary care centers to treat the poor free. All famous local doctors were asked to serve in the centers once a day. A night watcher of the city was swelling all over his body and his face turning into unhealthy yellow. Doctor Xue Xue, after seeing him and feeling his pulse, decided that his disease was not treatable. The patient went out of the door and happened to meet Ye Tianshi. Doctor Ye saw him far away from his sedan chair and asked, "Aren't you the night watcher? Your disease is due to inhaling toxic gas while smoking mosquitoes away. Take two doses of this medicine and you'll recover." Then he immediately made a prescription for him. Hearing what Ye said, Doctor Xue was greatly astonished and embarrassed, and grew jealous of Ye. He renamed his study "Saoye Zhuang" (meaning "Sweeping-the-leaves Room," as the character for "leaf" was the same as Ye's family name). In response, Ye Tianshi renamed his study "Taxue Zhai" ("Tramping-the-snow Room," as "snow" is homophonic with the Xue's family name). Both were famous doctors, and this was how their long running feud started.

From *Medical Cases Recorded in Lenglu*.

Editor's Note:

The story is quite enlightening, even if it was more anecdotal than factual. People in the literary circle always looked down upon each other because everyone considered himself the best. The same goes for doctors. Therefore, one needs to consciously reflect on oneself and learn from others.

【唐大黄】

【原文】

我邑唐介庵[①]先生，抱性[②]慈厚，於醫學深究南陽之旨[③]，各家亦能探討，中年後以用大黄著名。凡士大夫與窮巷僻鄉，遇有熱結不解者，必延唐大黄焉。于是乎先生之字，竟爲大黄之名掩矣。先生遇表證則汗之，虛則補之，寒則温之，亦何嘗執大黄而療人之疾哉？乃人遇欲下之證，延先生耳，非先生之偏用大黄也。

（選自清・黄退庵《友漁齋醫話》）

【注釋】

①唐介庵：浙江嘉善人，清代乾嘉年間名醫。②抱性：懷抱品性。③南陽之旨：指張仲景學説的含義。因張仲景的籍貫在南陽，故以“南陽”借代“仲景”。

【釋義】

我們縣城有位唐介庵先生。他性情仁慈，爲人厚道，在醫學上他精心研究張仲景學説的含義，對其他各家也能認真探討。中年以後，因善用大黄而著名，人們稱他“唐大黄”。不論是士大夫，還是窮鄉僻壤的百姓，得了熱結不解的病症，必是延請唐大黄治療。於是，先生的“介庵”這一名字，竟然被“大黄”一名所掩蓋了。其實，唐先生遇外感表證就用發汗藥，治虛證用補養藥，治寒證用温熱藥，又何嘗只拘泥大黄一藥來治療衆人的病呢？本來是病人患了須用大黄泄下的病證才來延請先生的，並不是唐先生偏用大黄一藥呀。

【按語】

《友漁齋醫話》八卷，是清代醫家黄凱鈞（號退庵）所著的一部醫話，刊於1812年。本書以筆記的形式，記録了作者在辨證治療、辨藥等方面的心得，内容廣泛，有一定的參考價值。

由於唐介庵善用大黄治疾，便得了個“唐大黄”的雅號。于是出現了凡“遇有熱結不解者，必延唐大黄”的現象，這正表明了病人對唐先生醫術的敬重和信賴。其實唐大黄並非偏用大黄，而是深究醫理，辨證施治：“遇表證則汗之，虛則補之，寒則温之，亦何嘗執大黄而療人之疾哉？”

金代大家劉河間有一穆姓弟子，也因善用大黄，人們尊之爲“穆大黄”，其真名早已被人忘記；明代大醫張介賓，因善用熟地，人們稱之爲“張熟地”；民國期間傷寒大家曹穎甫，因喜作梅花詩，人們便稱之爲“曹梅花”等。這些雅號、美名，是一種有趣的文化現象，它從一個側面反映了中醫藥文化的豐富多彩。

Doctor Tang Rhubarb

There was a doctor named Tang Jie'an in our county, who was kind and reliable. He elaborately studied the essence of Zhang Zhongjing's theory and explored thoughts of other doctors. By the time when he was middle aged, he had been famous for making good use of rhubarb root and rhizome (*Radixet Rhizoma Rhei*), so he was known as "Doctor Tang Rhubarb." High officials and common people in remote places alike went to see Tang Rhubarb, as soon as they suffered from febrile diseases. The doctor's original name Jie'an was almost forgotten, and he was universally referred to as Doctor Tang Rhubarb. Doctor Tang treated exogenous cold syndrome with diaphoretics, the deficient syndrome with tonics and cold with warm-natured medicine. His prescriptions were not at all constrained by the medicine rhubarb root and rhizome. It was just that Doctor Tang would use rhubarb root and rhizome effectively as a purgative rhubarb root and rhizome. As a doctor, he was really versatile and was not the least confined by the use of rhubarb root and rhizome..

From *Huang Kaijun on Traditional Medicine in the Youyu Study.*

Editor's Note:

Tang Jie'an got the nickname "Tang Rhubarb" because he was good at treating diseases with rhubarb root and rhizome. Patients worshiped and trusted his medical skills. Actually Tang Rhubarb didn't only use rhubarb root and rhizome. He probed in medical doctrines deeply and treated disease based on syndrome differentiation. A student of the great doctor Liu Hejian in the Jin Dynasty was also good at using rhubarb root and rhizome, thus was called "Mu Rhubarb" (as Mu was his family name). The great doctor Zhang Jiebin in the Ming Dynasty was good at using prepared rehmannia root (*Radix Rehmanniae Preparata*), and thus was known as "Zhang Rehmanniae" . The great doctor Cao Yingfu in the Republic of China (1912-1949) was good at treating typhoid diseases and writing poems about plum flower, and thus was called "Cao Plum flower". These elegant titles and names were all examples of an interesting cultural phenomenon in China, in which scholars and intellectuals were always associated with their expertise or hobbies.

【望色知溺】

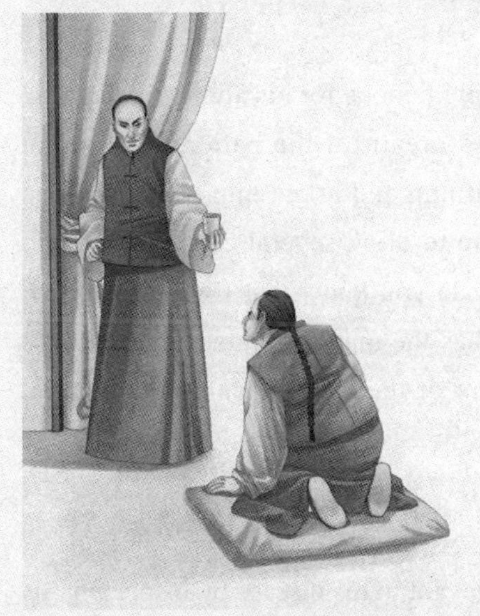

【原文】

青浦何元長①有醫名，尤擅望聞之術。有金山②人某來求診，元長曰："爾曾溺于水乎？"其人曰："然。"與之灌③，即愈。問："何以知其溺？"曰："望其色，黑而號④；切其脈，沉而牢。此陰寒内襲，是以知其溺也。"

（選自清 · 吳德旋《初月樓聞見録》）

【注釋】

何元長 (1752—1806)：名世仁，號澹安，又號福泉山人。今上海市青浦區重固鎮人。清代乾、嘉年間名醫。出於中醫世家，長於望聞之術，甚爲民衆所稱道。②金山：縣名。今屬上海市。③灌：飲酒。④黑而號：水色的標誌。

【釋義】

青浦（今上海市青浦區）何元長醫生很有名氣，尤其擅長望診和聞診。金山（今上海市金山區）有個病人來求診，元長診畢説："你曾被水淹過嗎？"病人説："是啊。"何元長讓他飲了幾杯酒，病就好了。病人問："您怎麼知道我被水淹過呢？"何元長説："看你的面色，有水色的標誌，診你的脈象，沉實弦長，這是陰寒襲及内臟，所以知道你是被水淹過啊。"

【按語】

吳德旋（1767—1840）：字仲倫，清代學者，江蘇宜興人。所著《初月樓聞見録》是清代筆記。成書於嘉慶二十三年（1818年）。

何元長通過望面色，一眼看出了病人的溺水之象，可見其望診技術之精妙。四診之中，望診爲首，古人多依據望診而定病之淺深。故今之爲醫者當重之！

Inspecting One's Complexion for Diagnosis

Doctor He Yuanzhang of Qingpu County was quite famous for his ability to diagnose based on inspection and listening to the voice and breath of the patients. A patient from Jinshan County came to see him. He examined him and asked him if he had been drowned. The patient answered, "Yes." He asked him to drink several cups of wine and then the patient recovered. The patient asked, "How do you know that I was drowned?" He Yuanzhang said, "Your complexion is dark and has the mark of water; your pulse is deep, solid, string-like and lengthy, which is the hint of the cold attacking the viscera. That's how I knew you've drowned before."

From *What I have seen and heard.*

Editor's Note:

He Yuanzhang knew the patient's past history relevant to his disease by inspecting his complexion. Inspection is the first step of the four-step diagnosis of TCM, the other three being listening, inquiring and pulse taking.

情志之疾

Emotional Diseases

【文摯治齊王疾】

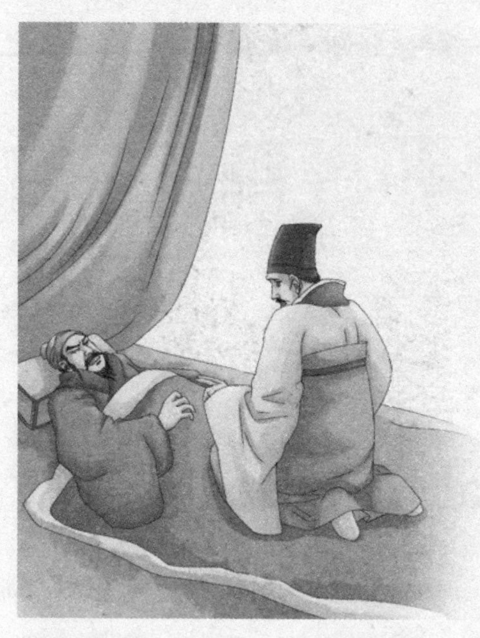

【原文】

齊王疾痏[①]，使人之宋迎文摯[②]。文摯至，視王之疾，謂太子曰："王之疾必可已[③]也。雖然，王之疾已，則必殺摯也。"太子曰："何故？"文摯對曰："非怒王則疾不可治，怒王則摯必死。"太子頓首强請曰："苟已王之疾，臣與臣之母以死争之于王，王必幸[④]臣與臣之母，願先生之勿患也！"文摯曰："諾。請以死爲王。"與太子期[⑤]，而將往不當者三[⑥]，齊王固已怒矣。文摯至，不解屨登床，履王衣，問王之疾，王怒而不與言。文摯因出辭以重怒王，王叱而起，疾乃遂已。王大怒不説，將生烹文摯。太子與王后急争之而不能得，果以鼎生烹文摯……夫忠於治世易，忠於濁世難。文摯非不知活王之疾而身獲死也，爲太子行難[⑦]以成其義也。

（選自《吕氏春秋 · 仲冬紀 · 至忠》）

【注釋】

①齊王：此指齊湣王。痏（wěi 偉）：癰疽之類，今之惡瘡。②文摯：宋國人，戰國時名醫。③已：止，病愈。④幸：寵愛。⑤期：約定日期。⑥不當者三：三次不如期應約。⑦行難：做難做的事。

【釋義】

齊湣王生了惡瘡，派人去宋國迎接文摯來治病。文摯到後，診視了王的病狀，對太子説："王的病一定可以治好；雖然這樣，王的病治好後，必定要殺我。"太子説："爲什麽？"文摯回答説，"如果不激怒大王，病就不能治好；如激怒大王，那麽我必死。"太子叩首下拜强請説："如果治好了大王的病，我與我母親拼死向大王争辯，大王必定愛憐我和母親，希望先生不要擔憂！"文摯説："可以。請讓我拼着一死爲王治病吧。"

文摯與太子約定了看病的日期，却三次失約而没有去，齊王本來就發怒了。文摯到後，不脱鞋就上床，又踩着王的衣服，問王的病况，王發怒而不講話。文摯又出言不恭重重地激怒王，王叱罵而起，病于是就好了。王大怒而不悦，要活活烹煮文摯。太子與王后急忙争辯，但不能改變王的决定，果然用三足鼎活生生地烹煮了文摯……忠於治世容易，忠於濁世困難。文摯並非不知治好了王的病而自己要死，只是爲了太子的緣故去做難做的事，成全太子孝敬之義罷了。

【按語】

《吕氏春秋》是由戰國末秦相吕不韋集合門客共同編寫的雜家代表著作。

這是用情志療法治疾的早期病例，給中國醫案史上留下了一個心理療法的典型范例。齊王生惡瘡，大概是由於思慮太甚，使氣血鬱結，結則蘊熱，熱則肉腐而成癰。文摯用“以污辱欺罔之言觸之”的激怒療法治愈王疾，正符合《黄帝内經》“怒勝思”的原理。而最終文摯被烹煮而死的悲劇，則反映了帝王的殘忍和對忠臣的不義。文摯的慘死，成爲古代醫學史上第一個以身殉職的悲壯事件。

Wenzhi Cured King Min of Qi[1]

King Min of Qi suffered from a malignant sore and sent for Wenzhi in the State of Song to come to treat the disease. Wenzhi examined the patient and told the prince, “The king’s disease is certainly curable, but he’ll certainly kill me after that.” The prince asked, “Why?” Wenzhi answered, “If the king is not irritated, he’ll not recover; if the king is irritated, I’ll certainly die.” The prince bowed to Wenzhi and urged him to treat the king, saying, “If the king is cured, my mother and I will risk our lives to defend you. The king will certainly show mercy on us. Please don’t be worried!” Wenzhi answered, “Fine, I’ll risk my life to treat the king.” Wenzhi and the prince set the date of treatment, but then Wenzhi deliberately broke the promise for three times, which angered the king. Finally, Wenzhi arrived. He climbed onto bed without taking off shoes and tramped on the king’s clothes. He inquired the king about the disease, but the king was too angry to answer. Then he irritated the king with rude words, which led the king to stand up and curse him. The king recovered after that, but was so enraged that he wanted to cook Wenzhi alive.

The prince and queen explained the reason, but could not change the king's mind. Wenzhi was cooked alive in a tripod··· Staying loyal and honest at times of peace and prosperity is easy, while being faithful in chaotic times is difficult. Wenzhi did what he did knowing the aftermath, to fulfill a doctor's duty and for the prince's filial piety.

From *Master Lü's Spring and Autumn Arnals*[2].

Notes:

1. King Min of Qi : 齊湣王 (ca.323 BCE–284 BCE or 300 BCE–284 BCE) was a notoriously incapable king of the northeastern Chinese state of Qi during the Warring States Period.

2. *Master Lü's Spring and Autumn Arnals* (《吕氏春秋》Lüshi Chunqiu): It is an encyclopedic Chinese classic text compiled around 239 BCE under the patronage of Chancellor Lü Buwei in the Qin Dynasty.

Editor's Note:

This is an early case of treating disease with emotional release therapy, a typical example of psychological treatment. King Min of Qi suffered from a malignant sore because the stagnation of his Qi and blood generated heat, making flesh rot and forming carbuncles. Wenzhi treated him with rude words according to the irritation therapy recorded in *The Yellow Emperor's Canon of Medicine*, but was finally brutally executed. This was the first recorded tragedy that happened to doctors who risked their lives for proper treatments.

【華佗留書罵郡守】

【原文】

又有一郡守病，佗以爲其人盛怒則差①，乃多受其貨而不加治②，無何棄去③，留書罵之。郡守果大怒，令人追捉殺佗。郡守子知之，屬④使勿逐。守瞋恚⑤既甚，吐黑血數升而愈。

（選自《三國志 · 華佗傳》）

【注釋】

①差：同“瘥”。病愈。②貨：錢財。加治：施治。③無何：不久。棄去，拋開

病人而離去。④屬：通“囑”。⑤瞋恚：怒恨。

【釋義】

又有一位郡守患病，華佗認爲讓那人大怒一番就會病愈。於是就大量接受他的钱財却不加以治療，不久又丟開病人離去，並留下書信辱罵他。郡守果然大怒，派人追捉要殺死華佗。郡守的兒子了解此事，囑咐追趕的人不要追捉。郡守憤恨得厲害，吐出數升黑血，病就好了。

【按語】

《三國志》爲西晉陳壽撰，共六十五卷，分魏、蜀、吳三志。

那位郡守大概是因爲患得患失，思慮過度，久則成病，而導致氣血鬱滯。華佗經過縝密的診斷，認准了病證，根據《黃帝内經》“思傷脾，怒勝思”的道理，大膽採用激怒之法，使郡守憤怒已極，結果吐黑血數升而愈。這一病例，與《吕氏春秋·仲冬紀至忠》中文摯治齊王疾一樣，都是典型的情志療法，對後世醫家産生了深遠影響。

關於此則故事，後人多有引述。北宋初年奉宋太宗之命編纂的古代小説總集《太平廣記》卷二一八，所記内容稍詳，可補《三國志·華佗傳》之不足。特録之於下：“魏·華佗善醫，嘗有郡守病甚，佗過之，郡守令佗診候。佗退，謂其子曰：使君病有異於常，積瘀血在腹中，當極怒嘔血，即能去疾，不爾無生矣。子宜盡言使君之愆，我疏而責之。其子曰：若獲愈，何謂不言！於是具以父從來所爲乖誤者，盡示佗。佗留書責罵之，守大怒，發吏捕佗，佗不至，遂嘔黑血升餘，其疾乃平。”

Hua Tuo[1] Cursed the Official

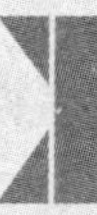

Once, a prefecture governor suffered from a disease. Hua Tuo thought that the governor would recover after getting angry and letting out the malignant Qi. Therefore, he accepted a great amount of his money and gifts but refused to treat him, leaving behind a letter full of cursing words. The governor was furious and sent people to arrest and kill Hua Tuo. Knowing the reason, the governor's son stopped the people after Hua. The governor was resentful, so much as that he spit out several sheng of black blood. He soon recovered.

From *History of the Three Kingdoms*.

Notes:

1. Hua Tuo (華佗 ?–208 AD) : As a famous physician in the late Eastern Han Dynasty (東漢 25–220) , he was famous for supreme surgery skills and for inventing methods of anesthesia.

Editor's Note:

The official got diseased due to the stagnation of qi and blood for worrying about personal gains and losses for a long time. Hua Tuo made a correct diagnosis and chose the irritation therapy according to records of *Inner Cannon of Yellow Emperor*. The official recovered after vomiting black blood. This is a typical emotional release therapy, which was often quoted by people in later generations.

【忽肥忽瘦】

【原文】

庾公造周伯仁[1]，伯仁曰："君何所欣説[2]而忽肥？"庾曰："君復何所憂慘而忽瘦？"伯仁曰："吾無所憂，直是清虛[3]日來，滓穢日去耳！"

（選自南朝·劉義慶《世説新語·言語》）

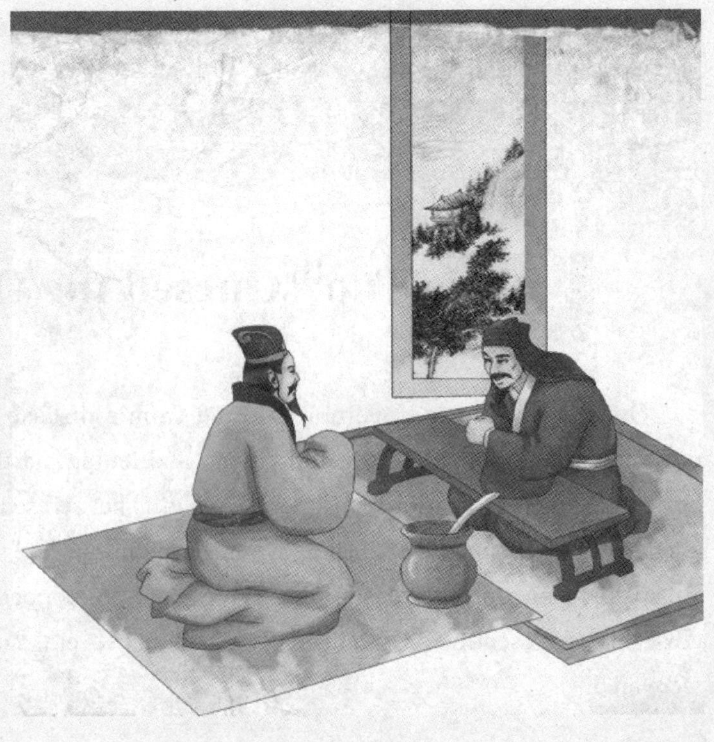

【注釋】

① 庾公：即庾亮(289—340)。字元規，又稱太尉、庾太尉、文康、庾文康。晉潁川鄢陵（今

河南鄢陵）人，明穆皇后兄。美姿容，好《老》《莊》，善談論。元帝時爲鎮東將軍，頗受器重，轉丞相参軍。明帝時，代王導爲中書監。成帝初，因其爲帝舅被任命爲中書令，執掌朝政。卒贈太尉，謚號文康。造：造訪，拜訪。周伯仁：周顗 (269—322) 的字，又稱周僕射、周侯。晋汝南安成（今河南正陽）人。少有重名，神采秀徹，累遷尚書吏部郎、荆州刺史。元帝即位，拜吏部尚書，遷尚書左僕射，執朝政。因嗜酒而屢有失，王敦起兵，被王誅殺。②所欣説：欣慰高興的事。説，同“悦”。③直：只。清虚：指清虚静泰之氣。

【釋義】

庾亮造訪周伯仁，周伯仁説道：“先生有什麼高興的事兒，一下子變得如此肥胖？”庾亮反問道：“先生有什麼憂煩的事兒，一下子變得這般消瘦？周伯仁説：“我没有什麼憂煩的事兒，只不過是清虚之氣一天天增多，滓漬污穢一天天减少罷了！”

【按語】

這兩位晋代名人的詼諧對話，雖然都是玩笑之語，但説明了人的身體健康與思想情緒密切相關的道理。

Gaining and Losing Weight

Once, Yu Liang visited Zhou Boren. Zhou Boren asked, “Have you experienced something pleasant? You have gained quite a bit of weight.” Yu asked in response, “Have you experienced something annoying? You’ve become emaciated.” Zhou Boren answered, “No, I haven’t. That’s because the clear quiet qi has increased in me and impurities have decreased day by day.”

From *A New Account of Tales of the World.*

Editor’s Note:

Though these two renowned scholars were joking with one another, the story indicates correctly the close relations between physical health and one’s emotional state.

看殺衛玠

【原文】

衛玠從豫章至下都[①]，人久聞其名，觀者如堵牆。玠先有羸[②]疾，體不堪勞，遂成病而死。時人謂看殺衛玠。

（選自南朝 · 劉義慶《世説新語 · 容止》）

【注釋】

①衛玠：字叔寶 (287—313)，又稱衛虎、衛君、衛洗馬。晉河東安邑(今山西運城)人，衛瓘孫。風姿俊秀出衆，善言玄理，名重一時，當時王敦、王導兄弟家聲譽很高，却有“王家三子，不如衛家一兒”的諺語。爲人寬容，無喜愠之色。因多病勞疾終。豫章：郡名，治所在今江西南昌市。下都：指京都建康（今南京）。②羸：瘦弱。

【釋義】

衛玠從豫章回到京都建康時，人們早就聽到他的大名，觀看他的人圍得像一堵牆。衛玠的身體本來就瘦弱，承受不了這種勞累，不久病重去世。當時的人戲稱：看死了衛玠。

【按語】

社會上致人於死之事固然多樣，殊不知還能“看殺人”。衛玠是一個風姿俊秀的謙謙君子，當人們聞其大名，竟然“觀者如堵牆”，以至於使這個已瘦弱多病的人，“體不堪勞，遂成病而死”。實在讓人扼腕！

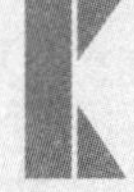

Wei Jie Exhausted by Spectators

When Wei Jie came back to the capital Jiankang from Yuzhang, people streamed to look at him because he was famous and said to be outstandingly elegant. Wei had always been quite weak, and now could not stand the burden of having to receive people all day long and being gazed at. He soon passed away. People at that time joked that Wei Jie was killed by too many spectators.

From *A New Account of Tales of the World*.

Editor's Note:

People die of different reasons, but this story is unusual. As a handsome noble man, Wei Jie was so famous that people visited him too frequently and gazed at him constantly, which contributed to his early death. What a pity!

【蟻動牛鬥】

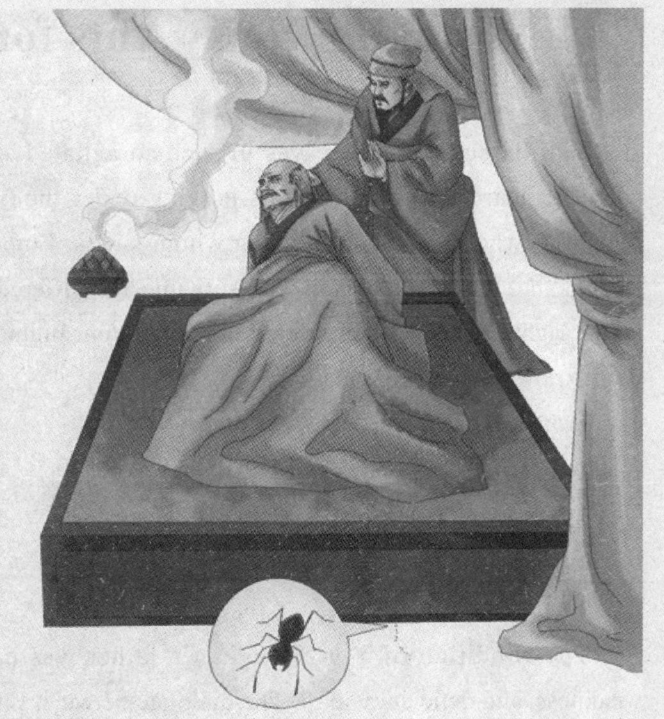

【原文】

殷仲堪父病虛悸[①]，聞床下蟻動，謂是牛鬥[②]。孝武不知是殷公，問仲堪："有一殷，病如此不[③]？"仲堪流涕而起曰："臣進退唯谷[④]。"

（選自南朝·劉義慶《世説新語·紕漏》）

【注釋】

①殷仲堪（？—399）：又叫殷荆州、殷侯。東晉陳郡（治今河南淮陽）人。善著文，能清言，與韓康伯齊名。歷任著作郎、長史，很得謝玄的賞識和厚待。後孝武帝召爲太子中庶子，領黄門郎。虛悸：心氣虛導致的心悸。②牛鬥：指群牛冲鬥聲。③不（fǒu 又讀 fōu）：同"否"。④進退唯谷：進退兩難。

【釋義】

殷仲堪的父親患了心悸病，聽到床下螞蟻的窸窣聲，以爲是群牛衝鬥。晉孝武帝不知是殷的父親，問仲堪："有一姓殷的，有這樣一種病，是嗎？"仲堪流淚站起來回答說："臣進退兩難，不知道該如何回答您。"

【按語】

殷仲堪父親患心悸病，聽到床下螞蟻的窸窣聲，誤以爲是群牛衝鬥。這是由於年老體弱，心氣大虛，心慌意亂而導致的幻聽現象。而孝武帝與殷公的對話，更讓人忍俊不禁。

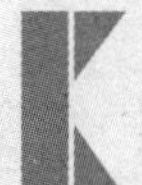

Mistaking Noisy Ants for a Bull Fight

Yin Zhongkan's father was in such an agitated and vulnerable mental state, that when he heard the sound of ants moving under the bed, he thought there was a bull fight somewhere. Without knowing whom it was, Emperor Xiaowu of Jin[1] once asked Zhongkan, "It is said a person with surname Yin suffered from such a (laughable) disease, is that right?" Zhongkan answered in tears, "Your highness, I'm in such a dilemma that I don't know how to respond."

From *A New Account of Tales of the World.*

Notes:

1. Emperor Xiaowu of Jin (晉孝武帝 Jin Xiaowudi, 373-396): He was an emperor of the Eastern Jin Dynasty (東晉 317-420) in China.

Editor's Note:

The condition of Yin Zhongkan's father was caused by his oldness, physical weakness, and deficiency in qi. The dialogue between Emperor Xiaowu and Yin was quite amusing.

【支道林感知音而死】

【原文】

支道林[①]喪法虔之後，精神殞喪[②]，風味[③]轉墜。常謂人曰："昔匠石廢斤於郢人[④]，牙生輟弦于鐘子[⑤]，推己外求，良不虛也。冥契[⑥]既逝，發言莫[⑦]賞，中心蘊結，餘其[⑧]亡矣！"却後一年，支遂殞[⑨]。

（選自南朝 · 劉義慶《世説新語 · 傷逝》）

【注釋】

①支道林：名遁，又稱支氏、支公、林公、林道人、林法師。晉高僧。本姓關，陳留（今河南開封縣陳留）人。一説河東林慮（今河南林縣）人。晉哀帝時應詔至洛陽東安寺，繼竺潛在宫禁中講法。支遁善談玄理，名震一時，時賢謝安、王羲之等皆與之交游。②殞（yǔn 允）喪：萎靡沮喪。③風味：風度。④"昔匠石"句：語出《莊子 · 徐無鬼》中《匠石運斤》的故事。匠石像風一般揮動斧子，砍削掉郢人鼻尖上的白泥，鼻子却一點也没有受傷，而郢人站在那裏紋絲不動任憑他砍削。後來匠石因郢人去世而放棄運斧。⑤"牙生輟弦"句：善於彈琴的俞伯牙遇到知音鐘子期的故事出自《列子 · 湯問》，成語"高山流水"即源於此。當鐘子期死後，俞伯牙認爲世上已無知音，終身不再鼓琴。本文引用以上兩個典故，意在説明高超的技藝還須有相應的對手配合。⑥冥契：指默契的知音。⑦莫：没有人。⑧其：或許，大概。⑨殞：死。

【釋義】

支道林在法虔去世後，精神萎靡，風度也日漸失去。常常對别人説："從前匠石因郢人去世而放棄運斧，俞伯牙因鐘子期亡故而終止彈琴，由自己此時的感受推及他人，的確不是虛言。默契的知音已經去世，談話没人能欣賞，心中鬱悶難以排解，我大概也要死了！"過了一年，支道林便溘然長逝。

【按語】

晉高僧支道林，因爲相交默契的知音法虔去世，精神萎靡沮喪，心中鬱悶難解，隨後便溘然長逝。從中可以看出他對朋友的深情，但從醫學的角度來講，更給人以深刻的啓示。

【Zhi Daolin Died after a Dear Friend's Death】

Zhi Daolin felt deeply lost and was no longer his normal self after the death of Faqian, his close friend. He told others for several times, that "the former Jiangshi stopped using axes after the death of Yingren, who deeply trusted him; Yu Boya stopped playing Chinese zither after the death of Zhong Ziqi, who understood him from his tunes. I could feel it exactly from my own experience. My friend who deeply and exactly knew me is now gone. No one could appreciate my thoughts any more. I'm probably dying too due to the mental depression and loneliness." One year later, Zhi Daolin passed away.

From *A New Account of Tales of the World.*

Editor's Note:

When Faqian died, his good friend, the monk Zhi Daolin felt depressed and soon died. Zhi harbored deep appreciation for his friend. His experience was of value to practitioners of medicine as well.

【王徽之哀弟而死】

【原文】

王子猷、子敬[①]俱病篤，而子敬先亡。子猷問左右："何以都不聞消息？此已喪矣。"語時了[②]不悲。便索輿[③]來奔喪，都不哭。子敬素好琴，便徑入坐靈床上，取子敬琴彈，弦既不調，擲地云："子敬！子敬！人琴俱亡！"因慟絶良久。月餘亦卒。

（選自南朝 · 劉義慶《世説新語 · 傷逝》）

【注釋】

①子猷：王徽之（？—388）字，又稱王黄門。晋琅邪臨沂（今山東臨沂縣）人。王羲之之子，獻之兄。官歷大司馬桓温參軍、車騎桓冲騎兵參軍、黄門侍郎，後棄官家居，以病終。任情放達，傲物慢世，性好竹，稱："何可一日無此君邪！" 子敬：王獻

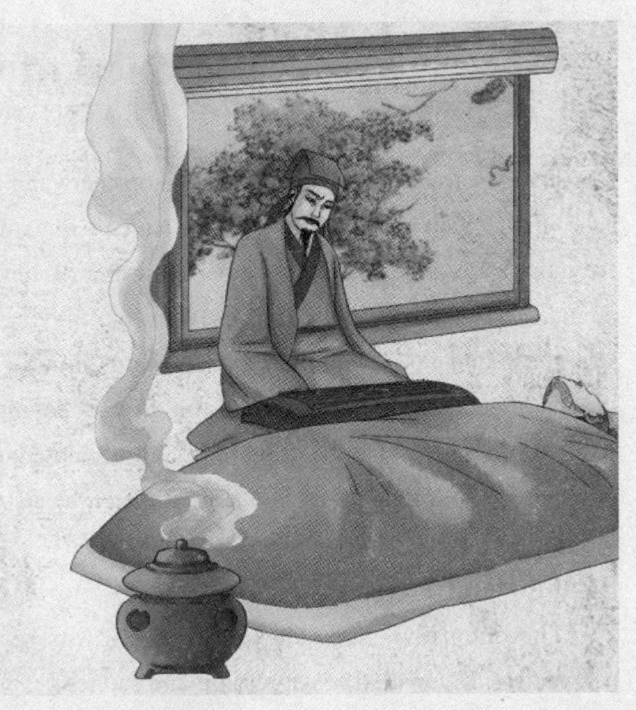

之 (344—388) 字，又稱阿敬、王令。王羲之之子，徽之弟。豪邁不羈，舉止嫻雅。官至尚書令，與王珣稱大、小令。病卒於官。獻之善丹青，尤工書法，骨力不及其父，而奔放豪邁過之，破古拙書風，啓張旭、懷素狂草之端，名重一時，與羲之並稱“二王”。②了：全。③輿：車。

【釋義】

王子猷（王徽之）和王子敬（王獻之）兄弟二人同時得了重病，王獻之先病故。王徽之問手下的人：“爲什麼聽不到一點子敬的音訊？這一定是已經去世了！”説這話時全然没有悲傷，便要車去奔喪，一點也没哭。王獻之平時一向喜歡彈琴，王徽之直接進去坐在靈床上，拿起獻之的琴彈了起來，琴弦怎麼也調不好，把琴扔在地上説：“子敬，子敬，你和琴都不在了！”于是痛哭以致昏了過去，過了好大一會兒纔醒過來。一個多月後他也病故了。

【按語】

王氏兄弟，情深意長，躍然紙上，甚爲感人！而從醫學的角度來看，本文同“支道林感知音而死”一樣，都屬於悲傷過度而致死的病例，有借鑒意義。

Wang Died of Grief

Wang Ziyou and Wang Zijing were brothers and both fell seriously ill. Zijing passed away first. Ziyou asked around, "Why haven't I heard anything about Zijing for a while? He must have gone!" He was quite calm then. Later, without grief and cry, he went to attend the funeral. Wang Zijing used to like playing Chinese zither. Wang Ziyou went straight in and sat on the bier, and took up Zijing's zither to play. He could not chord the instrument, so he threw it onto the ground, saying, "Zijing, Zijing, both you and the zither have gone!" Then he cried in grief and fainted. After a long while, he came back to consciousness. A little more than a month later, he also passed away.

From *A New Account of Tales of the World*.

Editor's Note:

The deep love between the brothers was really touching. From the medical perspective, Ziyou died of depression and sadness.

靖公巧施轉藥

【原文】

徐書記有室女[①]病似瘵，累醫不差[②]。聞靖公善醫，求診脈。公曰："子二寸脈微伏[③]，是因憂思之過，氣積於胸府中也。故病以膈氣而復苦勞疾。請示病實[④]，治之無差誤。"徐公曰："女子因睡中驚叫，言有蛇入腹中。細詢之，是夢見吞下蛇也。因此漸成病。"靖公曰："有蛇在腹中，須是轉下便差。某有斬蛇丹[⑤]，服之其蛇從大便中出。仍須貧道於側近守宿。"夜服其藥，果有小蛇下，女疾遂愈。

有好事者，詢之靖公。公密言："此非蛇病也。其女因夢蛇憂之過感斯疾。吾當治意[⑥]，而不治病。其蛇亦非自藏府中出，吾本只與轉藥[⑦]也。"

（選自唐 · 甘伯宗《名醫錄》）

【注釋】

①書記：掌管書牘記録的官員。室女：未嫁之女。②累醫不差：連續求醫治療，病不見好轉。差，同“瘥”。③二寸脈：寸脈主上焦病，左寸脈主心，右寸脈主肺。伏：指伏脈，主閉鬱。④示病實：説明得病的真實情況。⑤斬蛇丹：當時應急而假設的藥名。⑥治意：治心意中的病。⑦轉藥：指不直接治病而是轉移病人視綫的藥物。此指瀉下藥。

【釋義】

有一徐姓書記官的女兒尚未出嫁，面黄肌瘦，好像癆病，連續求醫却不見好轉。聽説靖公醫術高明，請來診治。靖公診完脈説：“你的女兒，兩寸脈象微伏而弱，這是因憂慮過度，氣鬱胸中所致，病是膈氣而又像勞瘵之疾。請你先説明得病的真實情況，再治療就不會出錯誤了。”徐書記官説：“我女兒因在夢中受驚，喊叫有蛇進入腹中。經仔細詢問，她説做夢把蛇吞下去了，因而漸成此病。”靖公説：“有蛇進入腹中，用藥瀉下來病就痊愈。我有斬蛇丹，能使蛇隨大便排出。但必須讓我在病人身旁守護一宿。”夜間病人吃了靖公的藥，果然瀉下一條死蛇來，徐公女兒的病就好了。

有好事的人，去詢問靖公。靖公便秘密地告訴他説：“這不是蛇病啊。徐公的女兒因做夢吞蛇憂慮太過而得此病。我是針對她的心理進行調治，而不是治什麼蛇病。這蛇也不是從她的臟腑中出來的，我只是給她瀉下藥物，解除她的思想顧慮而已。

【按語】

甘伯宗，唐代人，生平里籍未詳。曾編撰醫史著作《名醫傳》七卷，《宋史》稱《歷代名醫録》，後人稱之爲《名醫録》或《名醫大傳》。此書收集自伏羲至唐代名醫一百二十人傳記，是我國最早的醫學人物傳記專著。惜原書已亡佚，宋代《歷代名醫蒙求》等書有所引録。

那位書記官之女，因做夢有蛇入腹中，憂思太過而成疾。靖公虛擬所謂斬蛇丹，巧用轉移視綫的方法，解除了病人的思想顧慮，終於使情志憂鬱之病得以痊愈。靖公所言：“此非蛇病也。吾當治意，而不治病。”一語道出實情。這是典型的情志療法，正體現了“醫者意也”之義。

Jinggong's Effective Prescription

The unmarried daughter of an official with the surname Xu was emaciated from what seemed to be tuberculosis. Having received treatment for a long time, she still did not recover. Hearing of Jinggong's reputation, her father invited Jinggong to treat her. After the inspection, Jinggong said, "The pulse of your daughter feels weak and hidden. It is due to excessive anxiety and qi stagnation in the chest. Please tell me the real situation, and then I will make the correct judgment." Official Xu said, "My daughter was startled in a dream and shouted that there was a snake in her abdomen. After I carefully asked about what happened, she said that she swallowed the snake in the dream and then got the disease." Jinggong said, "She will recover if the snake could be purged down by drugs. I will prescribe the 'snake-cutting pill' for her to discharge the snake with the excrement, but you must allow me to stay and guard the patient for a night." During the night, the patient took the drug prescribed by Jinggong, discharged a dead snake and then recovered.

A gossipy person went to ask Jinggong about the reason. Jinggong told him, "The disease was not caused by the snake, but caused by the anxiety of swallowing the snake in the dream. I treated her psychologically, instead of treating the snake disease. The snake was not discharged from her body. I just prescribed the drug to relieve her worries."

From *The Biographies of Famous Doctors*.

Editor's Note:

The girl was so worried that she dreamed of a snake entering her abdomen. Jinggong made up the so-called snake-cutting pill to relieve her stress, and thus cured her disease. This excerpt is a typical case of the emotional release therapy.

【病怒不食】

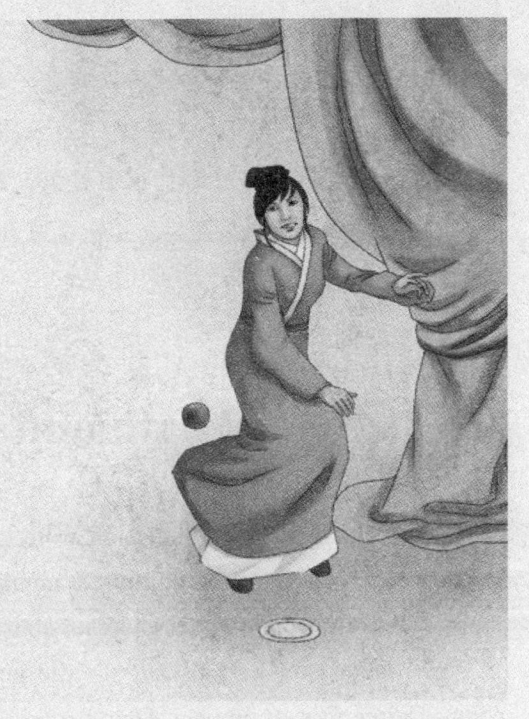

【原文】

項關令之妻，病怒不欲食，常好叫呼怒罵，欲殺左右，惡言不輟[①]。衆醫皆處藥，幾半載尚爾[②]。其夫命戴人[③]視之，戴人曰："此難以藥治。"乃使二娼各塗丹粉，作伶人[④]狀，其婦大笑。次日，又令作角觝[⑤]，又大笑。其旁常以兩個能食之婦，誇其食美，其婦亦索其食，而爲一嘗。不數日怒減食增，不藥而瘥。後得一子。夫醫貴有才，若無才，何足應變無窮。

（選自金・張子和《儒門事親・內傷形》）

【注釋】

①不輟：不止。②幾：將近。尚爾：還是原來那樣子。③戴人：即張子和。見"張子和擊木愈驚"條。④伶人：演戲的人。⑤角觝（jué dǐ 决抵）：即角抵。古時的一種技藝表演。類似摔跤。

【釋義】

項關令的妻子，因故患了暴怒之病，不思飲食，精神狂躁不安，常常好叫呼怒罵，揚言要殺左右之人，惡語不止。衆醫皆處方用藥，將近半年時間的治療，仍然還是老樣子。她的丈夫讓張戴人診視，戴人說："此病難以用藥治療。"于是叫來兩個妓女，各自塗抹丹粉，作伶人演戲狀，其婦大笑。次日，又讓她們表演摔跤，其婦又大笑。在她旁邊常安排兩個飯量大的婦女，誇贊其食物之美，其婦也就向她們索要食物，而進行品嘗。不到幾天，其婦怒減食增，不用藥而病愈。後來還生一子。當醫生貴在有本事，若無本事，怎麼能應付變化無窮的病情呢?

【按語】

《儒門事親》由金代張子和等輯著。十五卷。成於13世紀20年代。主要闡述運用汗、吐、下三法治病的理論和臨證經驗，並列舉了各類病症二百多例，用以説明其攻邪治法的療效。

項關令之妻，病怒不欲食。因病發在肝，怒氣冲逆，擾神明則狂，肝木克脾土過甚則不食。張子和使二娼塗丹粉，故做各種醜態，逗以戲嬉，使婦大笑。喜則氣緩，上逆之氣，得下消之喜氣，又誘以美食，故怒減食增，不藥而愈。《黄帝内經》云："怒傷肝"，"憂傷肺，喜勝憂"。喜爲良性情緒變化，可以抑制因鬱怒、悲哀等不良情緒所致病變。張子和的這個醫案，爲我們提供了一則典型病例。清代名醫魏之琇，在其所著的《續名醫類案》中，也曾引述了這一病例，並做了藝術加工。

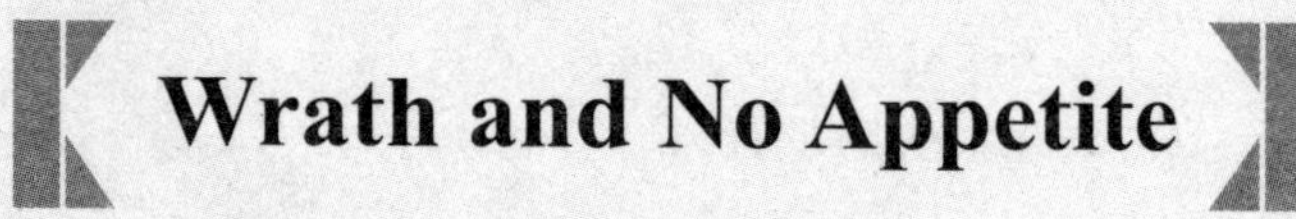

Wrath and No Appetite

Xiang Guanling's wife suffered from constant wrath for unknown reasons. Feeling irritated and uneasy, she could not eat anything and often shouted angrily at others. She claimed to kill surrounding people with abusive expressions. After receiving the treatment of many doctors for half a year, she did not get any better. Her husband asked Doctor Zhang Dairen to examine her. Dairen said, "The disease is hard to cure with medicine." Then he asked two prostitutes to dress up in a flashy and funny way to perform and amuse her. The woman laughed at them. The next day, Dairen asked them to do wrestling performance, and the woman laughed again. Then he asked two women with good appetite to keep her company and compliment the food constantly. Guanling's wife could not help but ask them for food to taste. Several days later, the woman was less irritable and gained some appetite. Then she recovered without taking medicine and later gave birth to a baby. One can see from this excerpt that a capable doctor has to be intelligent and adaptable, as he is likely to encounter patients with all sorts of problems.

From *Instructions on Fulfiling Fillial Piety*.

Editor's Note:

The wife of Xiang Guanling became too angry probably due to a liver disease and did not want to eat because the problematic liver suppressed the function of her spleen. Zhang Zihe asked two "actresses" to amuse her, which made her laugh. Delight relieved the anger and delicious food stimulated the appetite, which cured her without any drugs. Good mood is a benign emotion that counters harmful feelings such as depression, anger and sadness. This excerpt is a typical example.

【擊木愈驚】

【原文】

衛德新之妻，旅中[①]宿於樓上，夜值盜劫人[②]燒舍，驚墜床下。自後每聞有響，則驚倒不知人。家人輩躡足[③]而行，莫敢冒觸以聲，歲餘不痊。諸醫作心病治之，人參、珍珠及定志丸皆無效。戴人[④]見而斷之曰："驚者爲陽，從外入也；恐者爲陰，從内出。驚者爲自不知故也，恐者自知也。足少陽膽經屬肝木，膽者，敢也[⑤]。驚怕則膽傷矣。"乃命二侍女執其兩手，按高椅之上，當面前下置一小几。戴人曰："娘子當視此。"一木猛擊之，其婦大驚。戴人曰："我以木擊几，何以驚乎？"伺少定[⑥]擊之，驚也緩。又斯須連擊三五次，又以杖擊門，又暗遣人劃背後之窗。徐徐驚定而笑曰："是何治法？"戴人曰："《内經》云：驚者平之[⑦]。平者，常也。平常見之，必無驚。"是夜使人擊其門窗，自夕達曙[⑧]。一二日，雖聞雷亦不驚。德新素不喜戴人，至是終身厭服[⑨]。

（選自金·張子和《儒門事親·内傷形》）

【注釋】

①旅中：外出路途之中。 ②盜劫人：偷竊劫奪財物的人。 ③躡(niè 聶)足：放輕脚步走路。 ④戴人：即張從正，字子和，號戴人（约 1156—1228)，金元四大醫家之一。睢州考城（今河南民權西南）人。擅長汗、吐、下三法，後人譽爲攻下派代表。他曾爲金朝太醫，不久辭職。著有《儒門事親》十五卷（前三卷爲其親撰，其餘系弟子麻知幾、常仲明等整理而成）。 ⑤膽者，敢也：膽是主膽量勇敢的。 ⑥伺少定：等候病人稍微安定下來。 ⑦驚者平之：語出《素問·至真要大論》。 ⑧自夕達曙：從晚上到日出。 ⑨厭服：從心裏佩服。

【釋義】

衛德新的妻子外出旅途中，住宿在樓上，夜間碰上盜賊搶劫燒屋，因受驚恐而跌於床下。從此以後，一聽到響聲，就昏倒不省人事。家裏的人只得放輕脚步慢走，一年多病也不好。醫生們都按心臟病治療，什麼人參、珍珠、定志丸等，服之皆無效。張戴人診斷後說:“驚者爲陽邪,從外而入；恐者爲陰邪,從内而出。驚嚇是自己不知的緣故,而恐懼則自己知道。足少陽膽經屬肝木，膽是主膽量勇敢的。此病是因驚怕而膽氣受傷啊。”于是命令兩個侍女，把病人的手拉到高椅之上，在她面前放一小木凳。張戴人說：“你往下看這小木凳。”張即用一根木棒猛擊木凳，病人大驚。張戴人說：“我用木棒敲木凳，你爲何害怕呢？”等病人稍微安定下來又敲木凳，病人驚慌比前減輕。就這樣連續敲了三五次，又用木杖擊打門，又叫人暗地裏劃背後的窗户。病人慢慢地安静下來，笑着說:“這是什麼治法？”戴人說:“《黄帝内經》云：受驚嚇的人，要使之心情平静。”平，就是正常的意思。心情平静正常的狀態下，看見什麼，必定不驚。這天夜裏又使人不斷敲打她的門窗,從晚上直到天亮。這樣持續一兩日,即便聽到雷聲,病人也不驚恐了。衛德新素來不喜歡張戴人，自此以後，終身從心裏佩服他。

【按語】

張戴人以《黄帝内經》“驚者平之”之理，用循序漸進之法，使病人對當初驚嚇的聲音和情景漸漸習以爲常,而下視收神,安定神志,最終治愈了受驚之疾。清代俞震在《古今醫案按》中，也引録了這則病例，文字略有出入。

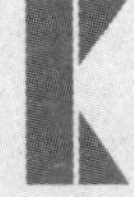

Striking Wood to Overcome Shock

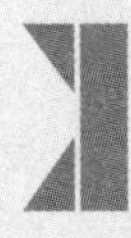

Once while out, Wei Dexin's wife stayed upstairs in a hotel. During that night, robbers came and burned the house. She was scared and fell from the bed. Since then, whenever hearing a sound, she would be startled and fell unconscious. Her family members had to walk slowly and cautiously around her. The situation lasted for one year and a half. Doctors all treated it as a heart disease, and prescribed ginsengs *(Radix Ginseng)* pearls *(Margarita)* and Dingzhi Pills, none of which worked. Finally, Zhang

Dairen was called for. Zhang examined her and said, "Shock was caused by an outside source, which is of yang nature, fear was from within and was of yin nature. One could not predict the source of shock but knew one's own fear. One's courage comes from a strong and robust gallbladder qi . The disease is caused by damage to gallbladder qi that originated from that shock." Zhang then asked two handmaids to hold the patient's hands and place her on a tall stool, with a small wooden stool in front of her. Having instructed her to look down at the wooden stool, he suddenly struck the stool with a wooden stick, which startled the patient. Zhang Dairen said, "I struck the stool with a stick. Why do you feel scared?" After the patient calmed down, he struck the stool again. The patient's fear reduced. Then he repeated for three to five times, struck the window with a stick, and secretly asked people to scratch the door behind the patient. The patient gradually calmed down and asked with smile, "What treatment is this?" Dairen said, "According to *The Yellow Emperor's Canon of Medicine*[1], people having been scared should maintain a peaceful mind." Peace comes from treating something as normal and routine. A person with a peaceful mind would not be startled under any circumstances. In the evening, he asked people to strike her door and window constantly until the next morning. In the next couple of days, he repeated the procedure and finally cured the patient's fear. She was not frightened even when it was thundering loudly. Though her husband never liked Zhang Dairen before, he greatly admired Zhang after this incident.

From *Instructions on Fulfiling Fillial Piety*.

Notes:

1. *The Yellow Emperor's Canon of Medicine* (《内經》/《黄帝内經》, Neijing/ Huangdi Neijing): It is generally believed to be compiled between the Warring States Period and the Han Dynasties; this collection is the earliest existing canon of TCM. It records systemized medical theories and practices, as well as ancient Chinese understanding of the natural and human world.

【因憂結塊】

【原文】

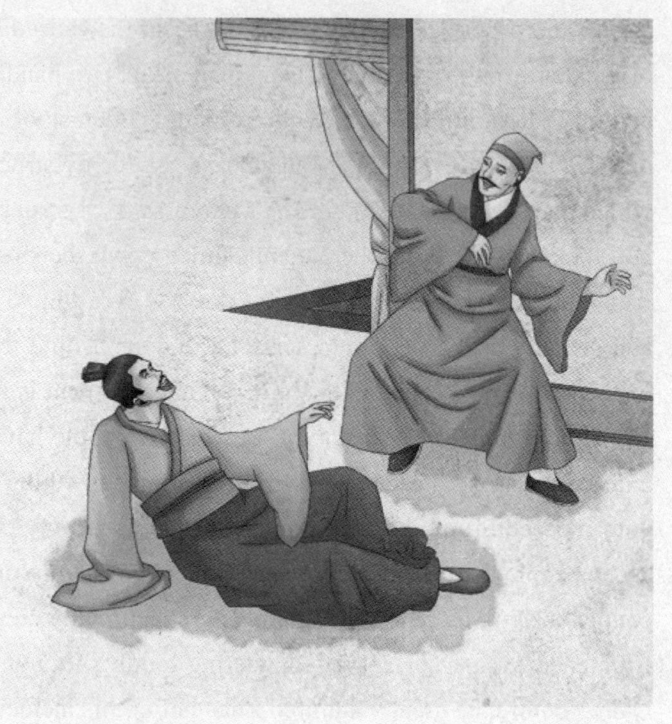

息城[①]司候，聞父死于賊，乃大悲哭之。罷，便覺心痛，日增不已，月餘成塊狀，若覆杯[②]，大痛不住。藥皆無功，議用燔針炷艾[③]，病人惡之，乃求於戴人。戴人至，適[④]巫者在其傍，乃學巫者，雜以狂言，以謔[⑤]病者，至是大笑不忍，回面向壁。一二日，心下結塊皆散。戴人曰："《内經》言：憂則氣結，喜則百脈舒和。又云：喜勝悲。《黄帝内經》自有此法治之，不知何用針灸哉？適足增其痛耳。"

（選自金 · 張子和《儒門事親 · 内傷形》）

【注釋】

①息城：今河南息縣。 ②覆杯：覆置的杯子。比喻心口像覆蓋着杯子一樣難受。③燔針炷艾：即火針艾灸。 ④適：正巧。 ⑤謔（xuè 血）：開玩笑。

【釋義】

息城縣司候，聽説父親被盜賊殺害，於是大悲痛哭。哭罷，便覺心口疼痛，且日增不止，一月多時間長成了塊狀，心口像覆蓋着杯子一樣難受，十分疼痛難忍。醫生用藥皆無功效，有人提議用火針艾灸，病人厭惡這種治法，便向張戴人求治。戴人來到，正巧有巫師在病人旁邊祈禱，於是便學着巫師的樣子，口中念念有詞，並加雜瘋癲狂語，來逗病人开心，至此病人大笑不止，回身面向牆壁。這樣一兩天光景，病人心下的結塊都消散了。戴人説："《黄帝内經》言：憂慮則心氣鬱結，喜悦則百脈舒緩平和。又説：喜勝悲。《黄帝内經》自有方法治療此類病，不知爲何要用針灸呢？這正是增加病人的痛苦呀！"

【按語】

憂則氣結，喜則百脈舒和。張戴人據《黄帝内經》"喜勝悲"之理，用戲謔之法，治愈了病人的因憂結塊之症。

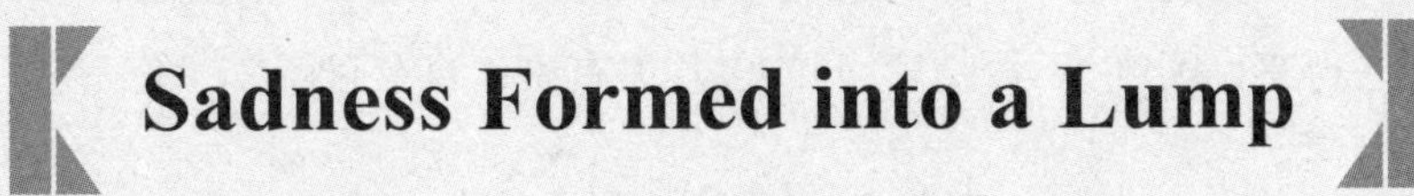

Sadness Formed into a Lump

A Sihou (an official rank) in Xicheng County cried in grief after hearing that bandits killed his father. After that, he felt more and more pain in his heart. After a month, a lump appeared there, making him suffer a great deal, feeling like a cup covering his heart. Many doctors treated him but they all failed. Someone proposed the moxibustion method with fire needles, but the patient disliked it and then asked Zhang Dairen to treat him. When Dairen came, he saw a witch praying beside the patient. He then imitated the witch and prayed with absurd words to amuse the patient. The patient laughed for a long time and then turned to face the wall. After one to two days, the patient's lump started to dissolve. Dairen said, "According to *The Yellow Emperor's Canon of Medicine*, sadness and worry lead to the qi stagnation in the heart, while delight soothes the vessels and help with circulation. It also says that delight can overcome sadness. This is all recorded in *The Yellow Emperor's Canon of Medicine*. Why would one use acupuncture or moxibustion instead? It will only increase the patient's pain!"

From *Instructions on Fulfiling Fillial Piety*.

Editor's Note:

Sadness causes stagnation of qi, while delight results in smooth and calm vessels. According to the recorded doctrine in *The Yellow Emperor's Canon of Medicine*, Zhang Dairen used the amusement method to cure the sadness and stagnation of the patient.

【丹溪掌擊相思女】

【原文】

一女子病不食，面壁卧者且半載，醫告術窮。翁[①]診之，肝脈弦出寸口，曰：“此思男子不得，氣結於脾故耳！”叩之，則許嫁丈夫入兩廣[②]且五年。翁謂其父曰：“是病惟怒可解，蓋怒之氣擊而屬木，故能衝其脾土之結，今宜觸之使怒耳。”父以爲不然。翁入而掌其面者三，責以不當有外思。女子號泣大怒[③]，怒已進食。翁復潛謂[④]其父曰：“思氣雖解，然必得喜，則庶[⑤]不再結。”乃詐以其夫有書，旦夕且歸[⑥]。後三月，夫果歸而病不作。

（選自元 · 戴良《九靈山房集》）

【注釋】

①翁：即丹溪翁朱彦修。見“朱謙葛雄”條注釋。 ②兩廣：指廣東、廣西。③號泣大怒：怒衝衝地放聲大哭。 ④潛謂：暗地告知。 ⑤庶：或許，可能。⑥旦夕且歸：很快將要回家。

【釋義】

有一女子得病不欲飲食，面朝牆壁而卧已經半年，醫生告訴病家無法治療，所以邀請丹溪翁前來診治。丹溪翁診察女子脈象，左手肝脈，弦長溢出寸口，便説：“這病是思念男子却又得不到，思則氣結於脾的緣故。”又問了問才知道，她許嫁的丈夫前往兩廣地區將近五年了。丹溪翁對她的父親説：“治此病只有激怒一法，因怒氣屬木，故能克化脾氣之鬱結，今應觸其心靈，使她怒氣暴發，鬱結之病纔能解除。”她的父親不以爲然。于是丹溪翁進入病人房中，朝那女子臉上連擊三掌，並責備她不應有外心。女子大哭大鬧，怒不可遏，怒後即能飲食了。丹溪翁暗地告知她父親説：“氣鬱雖然解除，但必使她歡喜，或許纔能使脾氣不再鬱結。”因而家中人騙她説：你的丈夫寄來書信，很快將要回家。三個月後，她的丈夫果然回來了，這女子的病也就再未發作。

【按語】

戴良（1317—1383），元代文學家，字叔能，號雲林、九靈山人，浦江（今屬浙江）人。 元亡隱居四明山。明太祖召見，託病固辭。著有《九靈山房集》，保存了一些著名的中醫傳記資料。因其未仕明，故稱元人。

這篇故事首先闡述了“思則氣結”的道理，接着以“怒勝思”之理而破其鬱結，然後又以“喜勝憂”之法進行調治，從而達到“喜則氣和志達”的目的。最終使患相思病之女得以痊愈。這一治療思路非常可取，至於朱丹溪是否真朝那相思女臉上連擊三掌，倒不必深究。

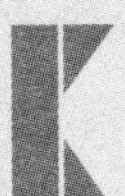

Doctor Zhu Cured the Lovesick Girl

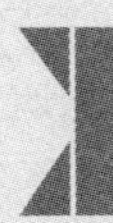

Once there was a girl, who suffered from a disease with no appetite. She lied on the bed facing the wall for half a year, and was diagnosed as being incurable. Then Doctor Zhu Yanxiu (aka Danxi Weng) was invited to examine her. Doctor Zhu felt the girl pulse on her wrist, and then said, “Her disease is due to qi stagnation in the spleen caused by lovesickness.” Then he learned that her fiance had left for the Liangguang District (Guangdong and Guangxi Provinces) for five years. Doctor Zhu told her father, “The disease can only be treated by the irritation method. The stagnant spleen qi could be overwhelmed by anger, which was of the wood nature among the five phases. Now we could try to irritate her to dissipate the stagnated qi.” The girl’s father did not take his words seriously. Then Doctor Zhu went into the patient’s room and slapped onto the girl’s face three times, blaming her for being unladylike and missing a man. The girl cried and shouted, feeling greatly insulted. She then started to gain her appetite back. Doctor Zhu secretly told her father, “Though the qi stagnation has been relieved, it will possibly recur unless she remains pleased.” Therefore, the girl’s family lied to her by saying that her fiance had sent a letter to inform that he was coming back soon. Three months later, he did come back. After that, the girl’s disease was completely cured.

From *A Collection of Works by Dai Liang*.

Editor’s Note:

The excerpt explains the cause and treatment of qi stagnation. The treatment is unconventional but reasonable in this case.

【得雨病愈】

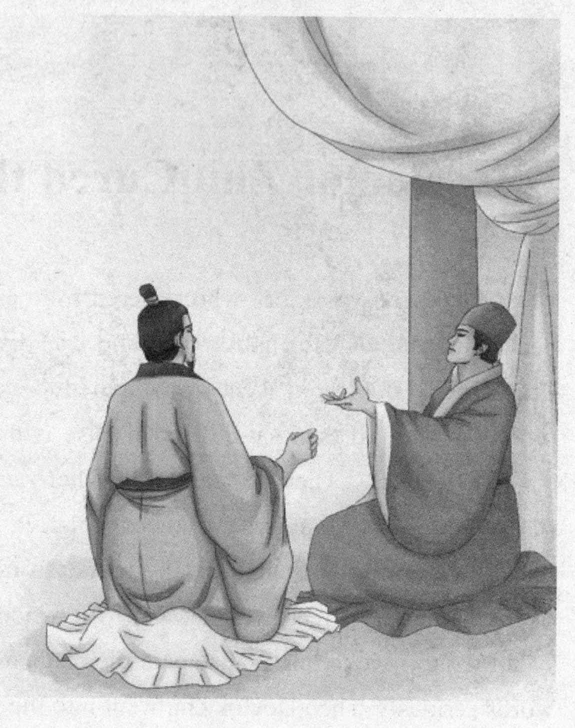

【原文】

昔者貴人[①]有疾，而天方不雨。醫來治者以十數，皆莫效。最後一人至，脈已[②]，則以指計甲子曰："某夕天必雨。"竟出[③]，不言治病之方。貴人疑之曰："豈謂吾疾不可爲邪？何言雨而不及藥我也？"已而[④]夕果雨，貴人喜，起而行乎庭，達旦，疾若脱去。明日，後至之醫來謁。貴人喜，且問曰："先生前日脈疾[⑤]而言雨，今得雨而果瘳[⑥]，何也？"醫對曰："君侯之疾以憂得之。然私計君侯忠且仁，所憂者民耳。以旱而憂，以雨而瘳，理固然也。何待藥而愈邪？"若是醫者，可謂得其道矣。

（選自明 · 方孝孺《遜志齋集》卷六）

【注釋】

①貴人：尊貴的人。②脈已：切脈完畢。③竟出：説完就走了。④已而：不久。⑤脈疾：診病。 ⑥瘳（chōu 抽）：病愈。

【釋義】

從前一位尊貴的人有病，天正一直不下雨。來治病的醫生有幾十個，都没有什麽療效。最後一個醫生來看病。切完脈，就掰着手指計算日子説："某個晚上天一定下雨。"説完就走了，也不講治病的方法。貴人對此懷疑説："難道説我的病不能治了嗎？爲什麽只講下雨却不提用藥給我治病的事呢？"不久，某個晚上果真下了雨，貴人很高興，起來在庭院中走動，一直到天亮，疾病就像一下甩掉了一樣全好了。第二天，最後來治病的那個醫生來拜見。貴人很高興，並詢問説："先生前天來診病時，講到下雨，如今得到雨果然病就好了，是什麽道理呢？"醫生回答説："您的病因憂愁而得。然而我考慮到您又信誠又仁愛，所擔憂的是人民百姓。因天旱而得病，由下雨而病愈，是理所當然的。爲什麼一定要依靠藥物治療才能好呢？”像這樣的醫生，真可以稱得上掌握醫道了。

【按語】

《遜志齋集》爲明代方孝儒（號遜志）作。共四十卷。

俗話說心病還須心藥醫。那位貴人患的病是“以憂得之”，天旱不雨，憂慮民生而成疾。醫生深知病人之心，診病切脈之後，並未用藥，只按甲子推算說了一句“某夕必雨”。不久果然下雨，病人大喜，憂遂解，病乃愈。“以旱而憂，以雨而瘳，理固然也”，何須用藥呢？正如文中所說：“若是醫者，可謂得其道矣”。

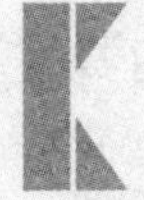

Recovery after the Rain

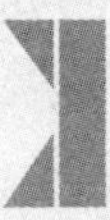

Once there was an honorable person who was diseased, and it had not rained for a long time. Dozens of doctors treated him in vain. Finally, a doctor came to examine him. After taking the pulse, he counted his fingers and said, “It will certainly rain soon in an evening.” Then he went away without saying how to treat the disease. The honorable man was bewildered, saying, “Has my disease become incurable? Why did the doctor only talk about raining instead of any treatment?” Soon, it rained indeed in one evening. The honorable man was greatly delighted and got up to walk in the courtyard until the daybreak of the next morning. By then it seemed that he had totally recovered from the disease. The next day, the doctor went to visit him. The honorable man was quite pleased and asked, “The day before yesterday, you came to examine me and talked about raining. Now I have recovered after the raining. Why?” The doctor answered, “Your disease was caused by deep worry. Knowing that you are upright and benevolent, I thought that what you worried about was the wellbeing of the people. The drought had kept you in deep concern, so raining would help you recover. That is a natural and effective treatment, more so than any medicine.” A doctor like this one is indeed a master of medical doctrines as he worked with the cause of diseases.

From *A Collection of Essays and Notes by Fang Xiaoru.*

Editor's Note:

The honorable man was diseased due to his concern with the drought and people's wellbeing. Knowing the cause of the disease, the doctor did not prescribe any drug after the examination. He just said that it would rain sometime in the future. Soon it rained indeed, which relieved the patient and enabled him to recover.

【葛可久擊案催産】

【原文】

一鄰婦，娠，將娩①，氣上逆，痛不可忍，就葛②治。葛見之，遽以掌擊案，厲聲大叱③，婦驚，産一子。葛慰曰："向見爾色青氣逆④，是腹中兒上攻，少緩不可救矣。猝然被驚，故即産也。"

（選自明 · 黄暐《蓬窗類記》）

【注釋】

①娩：生孩子。②葛：指葛可久，即葛乾孫(1305—1353)，字可久。元代著名醫家。長洲(今江蘇蘇州)人。其父應雷，以醫名世。葛公體偉，好擊刺戰陣之法，治病輒有奇效。著有《十藥神書》《醫學啓蒙》《論十二經絡》等。③大叱：大聲呵斥。 ④向：剛才。氣逆：此指胎氣上攻。

【釋義】

一鄰家婦女，懷孕要生孩子，忽然胎氣上攻，痛得忍耐不住，請葛可久先生治療。葛一見就用手猛拍桌案，並嚴厲地大喊一聲，孕婦突然一驚，立時生下一子。葛先生又安慰她說："我看你的面色發青，這是胎氣上攻的緣故，如稍微遲緩，就不可搶救了。猛然使你受驚，胎氣必然下降，所以纔立即生下孩子。"

【按語】

黄暐，名暐，字日昇，號東樓，吴縣（今江蘇省蘇州市）人。明代文學家，官至刑部郎中。所撰筆記小説《蓬窗類記》四卷，雜記舊事，上自朝廷典故，下及詼諧鬼怪之屬，無所不録。

元代名醫葛可久猛擊桌案，使正值胎氣上攻的孕婦得以順産，其奇驗如此，並非偶然。《素問·舉痛論》云："驚則氣亂，恐則氣下。"這一病例恰符合此理。且葛氏出自中醫世家，性格豪放，雄邁不羈，好擊刺戰陣之法，治病輒有奇效。這則病例也正體現了葛氏治法的特點。

Striking the Table to Help with Delivery

One day, a pregnant woman in the neighborhood was giving birth to a baby. Feeling the qi of the fetus forcing upward, she was in unbearable pain and could not deliver. Doctor Ge Kejiu was called for to treat her. As soon as Doctor Ge arrived, he suddenly struck the table and shouted loudly. The woman was startled and the baby was born quickly after that. Then Doctor Ge comforted her by saying, "I've noticed your face turning green, which was caused by ascending counterflow of fetal qi. It would have been incurable if delayed a bit longer. Being startled will help the fetal qi descend and smooth the delivery."

From *Assorted Notes by Huang Wei*.

Editor's Note:

Born in a medical family, Ge Kejiu was bold and aggressive. He struck the table to assist the delivery because the ascending fetal qi was restricted by the sudden surprise.

【喻嘉言嬉戲愈奇疾】

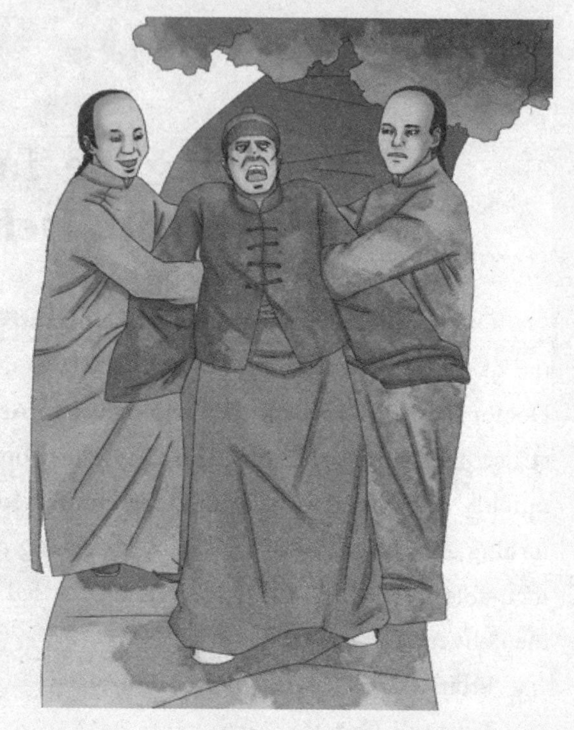

【原文】

牧齋[①]一日赴親朋家宴，肩輿[②]歸，過迎恩橋，輿夫蹉跌[③]，致主人亦受倒仆之驚。忽得奇疾，立則目欲上視，頭欲翻於地，卧則否。屢延醫者診治，不效。

時邑有良醫喻嘉言[④]，適往他郡治疾，亟遣僕往邀。越數日，喻始至，問致疾之由，遽曰："疾易治，無恐。"因向掌家[⑤]曰："府中輿夫强有力善走者命數人來。"於是呼至數人，喻命飫[⑥]以酒飯，謂數人曰："汝輩須儘量飽食，且可嬉戲爲樂也。"乃令分列於庭之四角，先用兩人挾持其主，並力疾趨[⑦]，自東則疾趨之西，自南則疾趨至北，互相更换，無一息停。主人殊苦顛播[⑧]，喻不顧，益促之驟。少頃，令息，則病已霍然矣。

時他醫在旁，未曉其故。喻曰："是因下橋倒仆，左邊第幾葉肝搐搦[⑨]而然。今扶掖[⑩]之疾走，抖擻經絡，則肝葉可舒；既復其位，則木氣敷暢[⑪]，而頭目安適矣。此非藥餌之所能爲也。"牧齋益神其術，稱喻爲聖醫。

（選自清 · 高士奇《牧齋遺事》）

【注釋】

①牧齋：指清初文人，牧齋先生高士奇，錢塘（今浙江杭州）人，字澹人，號江村。著有《春秋地名考略》《江村消夏録》《牧齋遺事》等。②肩輿：即二人抬的圈

椅式轎子。③蹉跌：失足跌倒。 ④喻嘉言：名昌，明末清初醫學家。⑤掌家：管理家庭事務的人員。⑥飫（yù 玉）：飽食。⑦疾趨：快走。⑧顛播：同"顛簸"。⑨搐搦（chù nuò 觸諾）：牽引，握持。⑩扶掖：架着胳膊。⑪敷暢：敷布暢通。即萬物生長化育之意。

【釋義】

牧齋先生有一天去親友處赴宴，酒飯後，坐着轎子回家。走到迎恩橋，轎夫不慎摔倒，使牧齋也跌仆受驚，就突然得了奇病。站着時眼往上看，頭往下栽，躺着就像正常人。多次求醫治療不效。

當時城中名醫喻嘉言，不巧正去外地治病，急忙派僕人前去邀請。過了好些天，喻嘉言纔到，問清致病之由，隨即便説："此病易治，不要害怕。"於是對管家説："把你家體壯善跑的轎夫叫些來。"管家立即喊來一幫人，喻嘉言一邊吩咐預備酒飯，一邊對轎夫説："你們儘量吃飽喝足，還可以盡情玩耍取樂。"隨後，吩咐轎夫立於院内四旁，先叫倆人攙扶牧齋快跑，從東跑到西，從南跑到北，前人累了，後人接替。這樣不停地快跑，牧齋感覺上下顛簸得很厲害，嘉言全然不顧，越發緊催快走。又跑了一陣子，纔讓停息下來，而牧齋之病已霍然而愈。

當時，其他醫生在一旁觀看，都不知道這是怎麼一回事。喻嘉言即對他們解釋説："這病是因爲牧齋下轎跌倒受驚，左邊第幾葉肝痙攣所引起。今攙扶病人快跑，就是爲了疏通病人的全身經絡，使肝葉舒暢；肝葉已恢復正常，則肝氣纔得以敷布暢通，所以頭部眼睛自然就安然舒適了。這種病不是藥物所能治療的。"牧齋聽罷，更加佩服喻嘉言的醫術高明，從此稱喻嘉言爲聖醫。

【按語】

本文表現了清初名醫喻嘉言先生卓越的醫術。他以嬉戲之法，疏通病人經絡，使其肝葉恢復其位，肝氣得以敷布暢通，而頭目安適，最終治愈牧齋先生之奇疾。可謂一件奇巧之事。

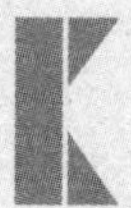

Strange Disease, Unusual Treatment

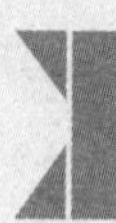

One day, Mr. Muzhai went to his relative's house for dinner. After the dinner, he took a sedan chair to go back home. When they were passing the Ying'en Bridge, a sedan-chair bearer fell to the ground by accident. Caught by surprise, Muzhai also fell, from which he developed strange symptoms. While standing he could not control his eyes from looking upward with his head dropping toward his shoulder, though he appeared normal while lying down. He saw many doctors but no one could cure him. Unfortunately, the famous local doctor Yu Jiayan had gone out to treat patients. He called for Yu and Yu did not come until many days later. Hearing the cause of the disease, Yu said, "This disease is easy to cure. Don't worry." He then told the housekeeper to find some strong sedan-chair bearers who are good at running. Doctor Yu then told the sedan-chair bearers "Have a good meal and have as much fun as you like." Yu placed the bearers on the sides of the courtyard and asked two of them to hold Muzhai's arms and run around in the courtyard. When the former two were tired, two other bearers would replace them. Fast running exhausted Muzhai, but Doctor Yu would not let them stop. After quite a while, Yu asked them to stop and have a rest. Muzhai soon recovered after that.

Other doctors watched the whole process, but could not understand. Doctor Yu explained to them, "Muzhai's problem was caused by his falling down on the bridge and being startled, which led to liver seizure on the left part. Asking other people to help the patient run fast was to dredge the channels all over his body and expand the liver lobes. The liver qi can only be regulated and unblocked after the liver lobes returned to the normal state. Then his head and eyes, which associated with the function of the liver, would naturally be back to normal. His conditions could not be cured by drugs." Hearing this, Muzhai admired Doctor Yu's superior medical skills, and thus called him the "Superb Doctor" .

From *Past Incidents Recorded by Qian Muzhai*.

Editor's Note:

The excerpt shows the supreme medical skills of the famous doctor Yu Jiayan in the early Qing Dynasty. He regulated patients' collaterals and meridians and restored the liver lobes, which smoothed the liver qi and finally cured the strange disease of Mr. Muzhai. This was really an unusual and legendary treatment.

【袖銀治疾】

【原文】

一鄰人手藝營生，積銀十兩，常置卧所。一日忽不見，遂病，醫藥終無效。先生[①]知其情，袖銀[②]如數，診脈時潛[③]置於枕席間。病人一旦復得，喜悦而病瘥。後皆知先生所爲，糾而還之，終無德色[④]。

（選自清・黄退庵《友漁齋醫話》）

【注釋】

①先生：指唐介庵先生。見"唐大黄"條。②袖銀：在衣袖裏裝銀子。③潛：暗地裏。④德色：讓人感恩報德的神色。

【釋義】

有一鄰居，依靠手藝謀生，積攢了十兩銀子，時常放在睡處。一天，銀子忽然不見了，於是卧病在床。請醫用藥，終無效果。唐介庵先生得知其内情，便在衣袖裏帶去十兩銀子，趁診脈之機，暗地裏放置在病人的枕席間。一天早上，病人發現銀子還在，喜出望外，病隨即痊愈。後來人們都知道這是唐先生做的好事，病家把錢還給他，而他始終没有讓人感恩報德的神色。

【按語】

情志過極，非藥可愈，宜用情志療法。《素問》云："憂傷肺，喜勝憂。"這位手藝人丢失了辛苦積蓄的"銀十兩"，憂思成疾；唐介庵"袖銀如數，診脈時潛置於枕席間"，使病人失而復得，喜悦而病愈。這正是"喜勝憂"的結果。值得稱贊的不只是唐介庵先生的高妙醫術，更是他那做好事而始終没有讓人感恩報德之色的高尚品質。

Curing a Disease with Hidden Silver

A neighbor of Doctor Tang Jie'an was a handicraftsman, and he usually put the ten taels of silver he had saved up beside his pillow. One day, the silver was gone. The handicraftsman immediately fell ill and could not recover for a long time. Hearing that, Doctor Tang hid ten taels of silver in his sleeves and secretly put it on the patient's bed while he examined him. Soon after, the patient found the silver, felt greatly relieved and recovered. Later, Doctor Tang's good deed was known and the patient eventually returned the money back to him. Doctor Tang, however, did not expect the money back or gratitude of others when he hid the silver.

From *Huang Kaijun on Traditional Medicine* .

Editor's Note:

Problems caused by excessive emotions cannot be cured by drugs and are best treated by emotional release therapy. The patient lost money and felt greatly upset and the doctor cured his disease by returning money to him. Both Doctor Tang's medical skills and his noble personality were admirable.

巧愈疑疾

【原文】

一人在姻家①過飲醉甚，送宿花軒②，夜半酒渴，欲水不得，遂口吸石槽中水碗許。天明視之，槽中俱是小紅蟲，心陡然而驚，鬱鬱不散。心中如有蛆物，胃脘便覺閉塞，日想月疑，漸成痿膈③，遍醫不愈。吳球④往視之，知其病生於疑也。用結綫紅色者分開剪斷如蛆狀，用巴豆二粒同飯搗爛，入紅綫丸⑤十數丸，令病人暗室内服之。又於宿盆内放水，須臾欲瀉，令病人坐盆，瀉出前物，蕩漾如蛆。然後開窗令親視之，其病從此解，調理半月而愈。

（選自清 · 俞震《古今醫案按》）

【注釋】

①姻家：指親家或有婚姻關係的親戚家。 ②花軒：廳堂前簷下的花草平臺。 ③痿

膈：胃脘痞塞。④吴球：字茭山，明代人。著有《諸證辨疑》《活人心統》《明志》等。其籍贯生卒不詳。⑤丸：製成丸。用作動詞。

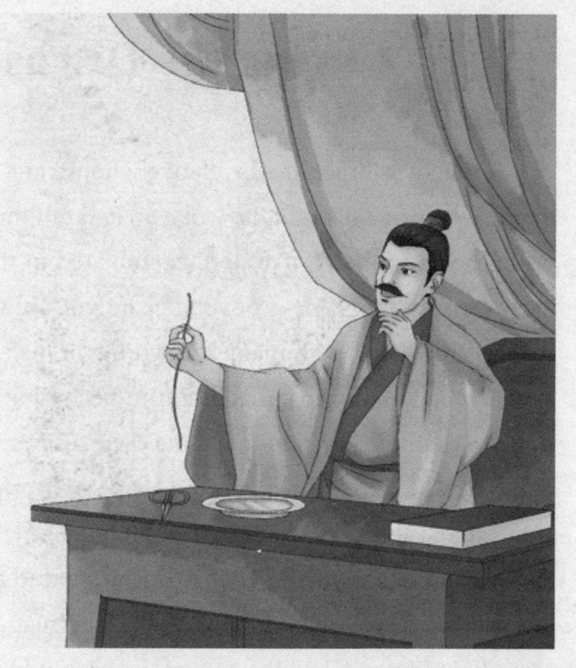

【釋義】

一人在姻親家裏飲酒過度，酩酊大醉，主人把他送到廳堂前的花坪涼臺上休息。睡到半夜，酒氣退而口渴，一時找不到能飲之水，無奈，就口吸石槽中的積水喝下約有一碗。天明起來，看見石槽中的積水生有很多紅色小蟲，心中突然一驚，氣鬱胸中，鬱鬱不散。心中疑惑，自覺腹内如有紅蟲蛆物。由此越想越疑，漸漸胃脘痞塞，成了心病，遍請醫生治療不愈。吴球先生前往診視，了解此病純屬因疑而生。先生把紅綫剪成小段，做成蛆狀，用巴豆兩粒，同米飯搗爛製成十多粒小丸，叫病人在黑屋裏把藥服下。又置備便盆放上清水，不大一會兒病人要腹瀉，急叫病人坐在便盆上，瀉出所服的藥物，在水中漂游很像紅色小蛆。然後開窗讓病人親眼看了看，這個人的病從此就好了。又調養半月就恢復了健康。

【按語】

俞震（1709—1799），字東扶，號惺齋，浙江嘉善人。清代乾隆間著名醫學家和詩人。自幼博覽群書，擅長吟詠，曾與兄弟等結同雅社。後因體弱多病，從金鈞習醫，得其秘奥。著有《古今醫案按》十卷、《古今經驗方按》等。

《古今醫案按》成書於1778年，按證列目，選輯歷代名醫醫案，上至倉公，下至葉天士共60餘家，1060餘案。所選醫案多出自江瓘《名醫類案》，對其他醫書屬立案奇法者，亦間采一二。俞氏在按語中，對各家的學術思想，褒貶分明，擇善而從。並結合自己的臨床經驗，析疑解惑。按語精闢，是研究前人醫案難得的佳著。

這則病例，同“杯弓蛇影”一樣，皆是因疑而生。因此，吴球巧用心理療法，疏其所疑，遠其所念，此病一舉而愈。

Curing the Disease of Suspicion

A man was drunk in his relative's house and was sent to rest in the balcony in front of the hall. During the night, he woke up and felt thirsty. Not being able to find any drinkable water, he had a bowl of water accumulated in the stone groove. Next day, he saw many red worms in the stone groove after he got up, which made him disgusted. He started to suspect that there were many red worms in his abdomen. The suspicion greatly upset his stomach and abdomen, in addition to becoming a severe mental illness. Doctor Wu Qiu came to examine him and found out the cause of his conditions. Doctor Wu cut red threads into pieces, making them into the shape of worms. He then made a mixture of purgative with the red threads, which he had the patient taken in a dark room. He also put water in the bedpan. After a while, the patient wanted to discharge. The doctor asked him to sit on the bedpan. The discharge looked like red maggots floating in the water. Doctor Wu let some light in and asked the patient to check it in person. After that, the man recovered and became healthy after half a month's good rest.

From *Medical Cases Past and Present*.

Editor's Note:

The problem recorded in this excerpt was due to stress and suspicion. Doctor Wu Qiu used a psychological therapy to cure the patient.

怒激少女發痘毒

【原文】

嘉言[①]往鄉，舟過一村落，見一少女子沙際搗[②]衣。注視久之，忽呼停棹[③]，命一壯僕曰："汝登岸潛近[④]女身，亟從後抱住，非我命無釋手。"僕如其言，女怒且罵，大呼其父母出，欲毆之。嘉言徐諭[⑤]曰："我喻某，適見此女將攖[⑥]危症，故明救[⑦]，非惡意也。"女父母素聞喻名，乃止。喻問曰："汝女未痘乎？"曰："然。"喻曰："數日將發悶痘，萬無可救，吾所以令僕激其怒者，乘其未發，先泄其肝火，使勢少衰，後日藥力可施也。至期，可於北城外某處來取藥，無遲。”

越數日，忽有夜叩喻門者，則向[8]所遇村中少女之父也。言女得熱疾，煩躁不寧之狀。喻問：“膚間有痘影否？”曰：“不但現影，且現形。”喻慰之曰：“汝女得生矣。”乃俾[9]以托裏之劑，其痘發透。此女得無恙。

（選自清 · 高士奇《牧齋遺事》）

【注釋】

①嘉言：即喻嘉言。見《喻嘉言一針救二命》注釋。 ②沙際：水邊。 搗：砸。古時洗衣多用棒槌在石板上捶打。 ③棹（zhào 趙）：划船用的槳。 ④潛近：暗中靠近。 ⑤徐諭：慢慢地告知。 ⑥將攖（yīng 英）：將要得病。 ⑦明救：公然用此法相救。 ⑧向：以前。⑨俾：使用。

【釋義】

喻嘉言先生乘船往鄉村去，路經一個村莊時，見一少女在河邊洗衣。嘉言定睛看了好久，突然喊聲停船，他對一名强壯的僕人說：“你登上岸去，暗地裏接近少女，從後面急忙抱住她，聽我說話你再放手。”僕人照此去做，那少女憤怒掙扎，大聲喊罵，並高聲招呼父母，她父母出來一看，急欲毆打僕人。嘉言慢慢地解釋說：“我是喻嘉言，剛才看見你的女兒將有大病臨身，因而公然用此法相救，並非惡意呀！”少女的父母素日聽說喻嘉言的大名，便即刻放手。喻嘉言問道：“你的女兒還没出過痘吧？”回答說：“是啊。”嘉言說：“近幾天你的女兒要生悶痘，將無法救治，所以我叫僕人激發她的怒氣，是爲了在悶痘未出之前，先發泄她的肝火，使病勢减弱，再用藥就容易收效了。等你女兒發病時，到城北我家取藥，不能耽誤時間。”

過了幾天，突然有人深夜前來敲喻嘉言的門，正是先前下鄉遇見的那位少女的父親。一進門就說：他女兒得了熱病，出現煩躁不安的情形。喻嘉言問：“皮膚間見到痘的影子了嗎？”回答說：“不但出現痘的影子，並且顯露痘的形狀了。”喻嘉言安慰他說：“你的女兒有救了。”於是使用托裏透表的藥物治療，少女服藥後，痘毒透發，不久病就痊愈了。

【按語】

這則妙趣橫生的故事，展現了一代名醫喻嘉言的大師風采。他那望診如神的診病技術和豐富多彩的臨證經驗，出神入化，讓人嘆服。

Pox Eruption Due to Irritation

When Doctor Yu Jiayan was once on his way to the countryside by boat, he saw a girl washing clothes on the riverside. He watched her from a distance for a while, stopped the boat and told a strong servant to approach the girl secretly and hold her until the doctor asked him to stop. The servant followed his words. The girl struggled angrily while shouting, scolding and calling her parents. Her parents came out to beat the servant up. Jiayan explained to the parents who he was, and said "I noticed that your daughter would fall seriously ill, and saved her with this method. I did not have any ill intention." Having heard of Yu Jiayan's reputation, the girl's parents immediately released the servant. Doctor Yu asked if the girl had had pox before, and was told she had not. Doctor Yu then explained, "She would have developed the incurable type of hidden pox soon, so I asked the servant to irritate her to dissipate heat in her liver. Now her disease will get more manageable and curable. Go find me in the northern town to get the medicine immediately after the pox appears."

Several days later, someone knocked on Doctor Yu's door in the middle of the night. It was the father of the girl, who said that his daughter had suffered from the febrile disease and become restless. Doctor Yu asked, "Is there anything appearing like poxes on the skin?" The father answered, "There clearly has been appearance of poxes." Doctor Yu comforted him by saying, "Your daughter is curable now." Then he prescribed the drugs to expel the internal toxic elements. The girl took the drug, which prompted her poxes to erupt, and she soon recovered.

From *Past Incidents Recorded by Qian Muzhai*..

Editor's Note:

This excerpt vividly demonstrates the demeanor and professional capabilities of the famous doctor Yu Jiayan. He could see a potential medical problem by inspection, and gave step-by-step instruction on how to treat the patient. In this way, he saved the girl's life.

【恐嚇愈狂舉】

【原文】

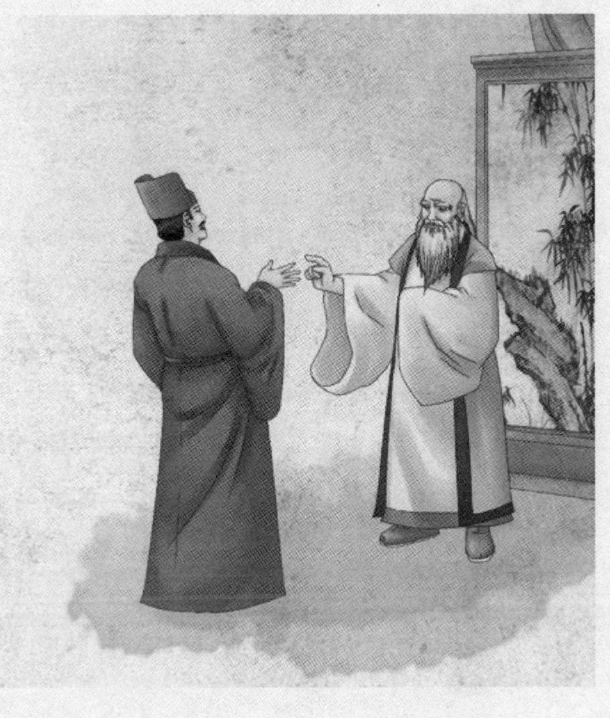

明末，高郵[①]有袁體庵者，神醫也。有舉子舉於鄉[②]，喜極，發狂,笑不止。求體庵診之,驚曰:“疾不可爲[③]矣！不以數旬[④]矣！子宜急歸，遲恐不及也。若道過鎮江[⑤]，必更求何氏診之。”遂以一書寄何。其人至鎮江而疾已愈，以書致何。何以書示[⑥]其人，曰：“某某喜極而狂，喜則心竅開張而不可復合，非藥石之所能治也。故動以危苦之心[⑦]，懼之以死，令其憂愁抑鬱，則心竅閉，至鎮江當已愈矣。”其人見之，北面再拜[⑧]而去。

（選自清 · 劉獻廷《廣陽雜記》[⑨]）

【注釋】

①高郵：縣名。在今江蘇省中部。 ②舉子：被選舉應試的讀書人。舉於鄉：即在鄉試中考中舉人。 ③爲：治。 ④不以數旬：活不了幾十天了。 ⑤鎮江：即江蘇省鎮江一帶。 ⑥示：給人看。 ⑦危苦之心：恐懼苦惱的心情。 ⑧再拜：古代的一種禮節，即先後拜兩次，表示禮節隆重。 ⑨《廣陽雜記》：見《螃蟹解漆毒》注釋。

【釋義】

明代末年，江蘇高郵有位名醫叫袁體庵，治病如神。曾經有一讀書人，考中了舉人，歡喜非常，因而病狂，大笑不止。于是請求袁體庵先生診治，袁體庵得知病情，便裝作大吃一驚的樣子對舉人說：“你的病情危險極了，活不了幾十天了，你應趕快回家，如再耽誤時間，恐怕走不到家了。”又說：“你路過鎮江，必須再求何醫生給你治療，或許有辦法能治好。”說罷立即寫了信，並囑咐把信交給何醫生。這位舉人抱着恐懼苦惱的心情，來到鎮江，他的笑狂之病已痊愈，於是舉人把袁體庵的書信送交何醫生。何醫生拆信一看，又遞給舉人，信上寫道："某某舉人因爲過度歡喜而心傷病狂，由於心神過於激動，以致心神不得安寧，此病不是藥物能够治好的。所以我用危險痛苦來恫嚇他，使他懼怕死亡，憂愁抑鬱，則心神收斂自然安寧，預計走到鎮江，舉人的病就應該痊愈了。"舉人看完此信深爲感謝，便面朝北方先後拜了兩次，就回家去了。

【按語】

劉獻廷，字繼莊，一字君賢，別號廣陽子。直隸大興（今北京）人，清初學者。清順治五年（1648年）生，康熙三十四年（1695年）卒，年48歲。劉獻廷學識淵博，且深明醫道，有所創見。《廣陽雜記》共五卷，此書不編類，是隨手記録之作。內容涉及"禮樂、象緯、醫藥、書數、法律、農桑、火攻、器制"等，所記翔實可信。

袁體庵以危苦之心，懼之以死的恫嚇之法，治愈了舉人的喜極而狂之疾。這正符合《黄帝內經》"喜傷心，恐勝喜"的治療法則，耐人尋味。

Ecstasy Cured by Intimidation

In the late Ming Dynasty, a famous doctor Yuan Ti'an lived in Gaoyou county of Jiangsu Province. He had always been effective in his treatment of numerous patients. Once there was a scholar, who was so excited about passing the provincial level of the civil service examination that he was overcome by ecstasy and could not stop laughing. Then he was sent to see Doctor Yuan Ti'an, who examined him and pretended to be deeply concerned, telling him "You're in danger now and could only live for dozens of days. You should return home soon. If not, you would not have a chance to see home again." He then added, "When you pass Zhenjiang, you should seek for a treatment from Doctor He. Maybe he will cure you." Then Doctor Yuan wrote a letter for the scholar to send to Doctor He.

When the scholar reached Zhenjiang, he had returned to his normal state due to his deep fear and worry. He handed over the letter of Yuan Ti'an to Doctor He. Doctor He passed the letter back to the scholar. It said in the letter, "This scholar was overjoyed and lost his sanity due to heart damage. Drugs could not cure this disease. Therefore, I intimidated him with an incurable disease. This would depress and upset him and then calm down his mind. He should have recovered by the time when he arrives at Zhenjiang." The scholar felt quite grateful after reading the letter, bowed twice facing the north and then went back home.

From *Miscellaneous Essays and Notes by Liu Xianting*.

Editor's Note:

Yuan Ti'an cured the scholar's disease by frightening him because the disease was due to extreme excitement and joy.

【佯爲郵語止笑症】

【原文】

先達[①]李其姓，歸德府鹿邑[②]人也。世爲農家，癸卯獲雋於鄉[③]。伊[④]父以喜故，失聲大笑。及春舉進士[⑤]，其笑彌甚。歷十年，擢諫垣[⑥]，遂成痼疾。初猶間發，後宵旦不能休。大諫甚憂之，從容語太醫院某，因得所授。命家人紿[⑦]乃父云："大諫已殁。"乃父慟絶，幾殞[⑧]。如是者十日，病漸瘳。佯爲郵語[⑨]云："大諫治以趙大夫，絶而復蘇。"李因不悲，而笑證永不作矣。蓋醫者意也，過喜則傷，濟以悲而乃和，技進乎道矣。

（選自清 · 陳尚古《簪雲樓雜説》）

【注釋】

①先達：舊時尊稱有地位、有聲望的前輩爲先達。②歸德府：府名，治所在今河南省商丘市。鹿邑：縣名，在今河南省東南部。③獲雋於鄉：鄉試得中舉人。雋，通"俊"，才智過人。④伊：他。⑤進士：凡舉人經會試考中者爲貢士，由貢士經殿試賜出身者爲進士。⑥擢（zhuó 濁）諫垣：提拔爲諫院的官員。⑦紿（dài 待）：欺騙。⑧幾殞：將近死亡。⑨佯爲郵語：謊稱來信説。

【釋義】

有一先賢李某，是歸德府鹿邑縣人。世代爲農，癸卯年間鄉試得中舉人。他的父親因爲高興，禁不住放聲大笑。到了春天，李某又考中進士，他父親笑得更加厲害了。過了十年，李某又提升爲諫院的官員，他父親的大笑就成了難以治愈的頑症。起初是大笑時斷時續地發作，後來就從早到晚不能停止了。李某爲此非常憂慮，順便把這個情況告訴了太醫院的一位御醫。御醫授意李某，就讓家中人欺騙他父親説："大諫李某得病已經死了。"他父親聽了轉喜爲悲，痛哭欲絶，幾乎昏死過去。就這樣經過了十天，他父親的笑症逐漸地好了。家中人又謊言李某來信説他的病得到御醫趙大夫的治療，死而復生。他父親也就不再悲傷，從此笑症再没發作。醫就是意呀。喜太過則傷心，故濟之以悲才能平和。醫技是合乎道的。

【按語】

陳尚古，字彦樸，江蘇長洲（今蘇州）人，生卒年不詳。清代學者。精於繪畫，善山水。所著《簪雲樓雜説》系筆記小説，讀來饒多意趣。

《素問·五運行大論》説："喜傷心，恐勝喜。"此病因過喜則傷心，故濟之以悲乃平和，佯爲鄄語而治愈了李父的狂笑之症。此亦即"醫者意也"之謂也。

A Lie that Cured Gelotolepsy

There was a person with the surname of Li, a native of Luyi County of Gui De Prefecture. His family had been engaged in farming for generations. During the Guimao year, he passed the provincial level of the civil service examination. His father was so delighted that he could not help laughing aloud. The next spring, Li passed the highest level of the civil service examination, which made his father laugh more loudly and frequently. Ten years later, Li was promoted to a position in Jianyuan, a high-level government office that supervised officials' behaviors. By then the father's laughing had become an incurable disease. He laughed loudly at intervals in the beginning, but by this point, he could not stop and laughed all day long.

Li was quite worried, so he asked a doctor who treated the royalty and high officials. The doctor asked Li to tell his family members to lie to his father by saying that Li died of a disease. Hearing that, his father was greatly saddened, cried desperately and nearly fainted. Ten days later, his father completely recovered from the gelotolepsy. His family members then told him that Li had been cured by imperial doctor Zhao and had just revived. The father did not grieve any more but never suffered from gelotolepsy again. To treat the patient, one needs to know what the disease was. Too much happiness hurts the heart, which could only be offset by sadness. Medical doctrines are in accordance with the natural laws and reason.

From *Miscellaneous Essays Written on Zanyun House*.

Editor's Note:

Excessive joy damaged the heart and caused the disease. Thus, a bad news was fabricated to make the patient sad and help him calm down.

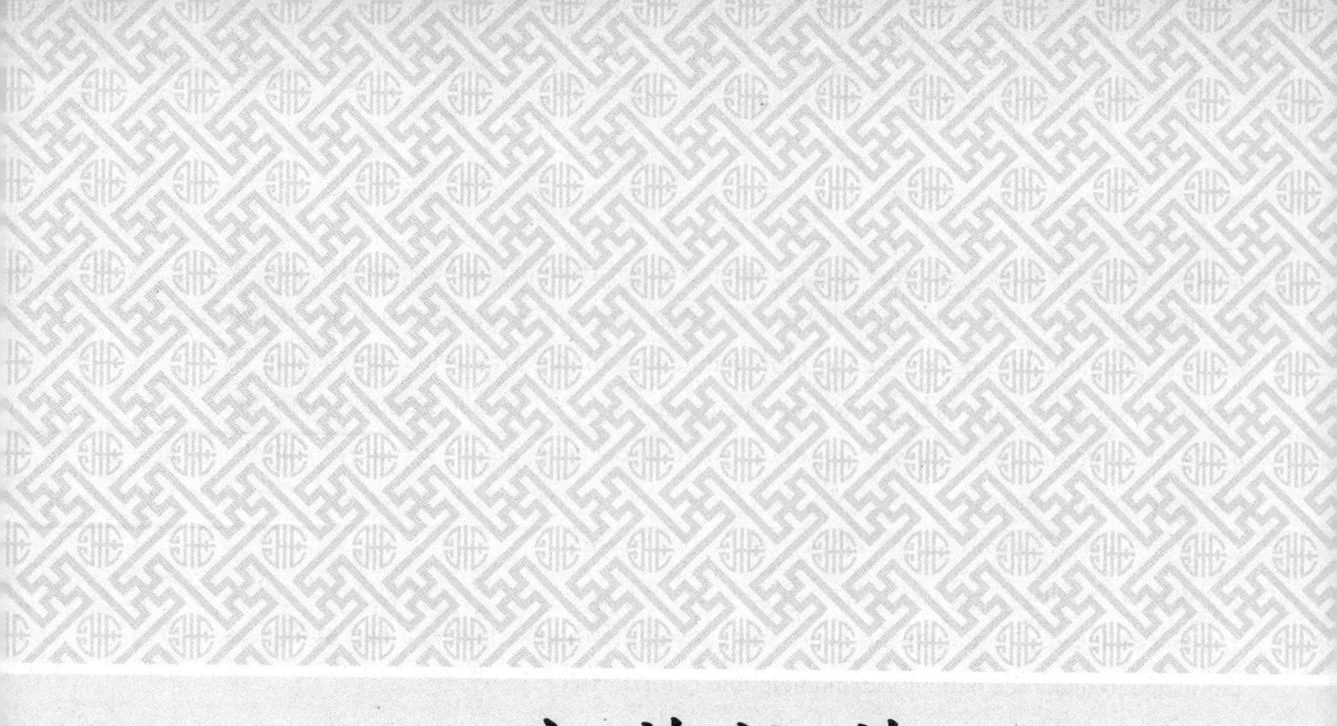

本草拾萃

Finely Selected Notes on Herbal Medicine

【遠志小草】

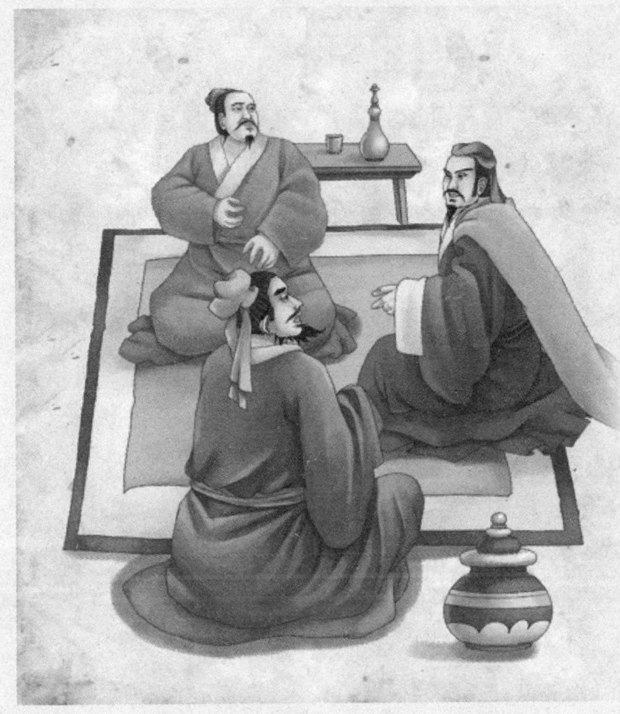

【原文】

謝公①始有東山之志，後嚴命屢臻②，勢不獲已，始就桓公③司馬。于時人有餉④桓公藥草，中有遠志。公取以問謝："此藥又名小草，何一物而有二稱？"謝未即答。時郝隆⑤在坐，應聲答曰："此甚易解。處則爲遠志，出則爲小草。"謝甚有愧色。桓公目謝而笑曰"郝參軍此過乃不惡⑥，亦極有會。"

（選自南朝 · 劉義慶《世説新語 · 排調》）

【注釋】

①謝公：即謝安(320—385)，字安石，又稱太傅、謝太傅。晉陳郡陽夏（今河南太康縣）人。他風流瀟灑，少負重名。謝安能暢談、善行書、好音樂、喜宴游、有雅量。苻堅南侵，謝安爲征討大都督，派謝玄等破敵於淝水。病逝後，追贈太傅，謚文靖。②嚴命屢臻：朝廷徵召的命令多次下達。③桓公：即桓温(312—373)，字元子，又稱桓宣城、桓宣武、桓大司馬、大將軍。晉代譙國龍亢（今安徽懷遠縣西北）人。晉攻伐前秦時，桓温攻破姚襄，威權大盛，官至大司馬。後來準備篡晉自立，未果而死，謚宣武侯。後其子桓玄篡位，追尊其爲宣武皇帝。④餉：贈送。⑤郝隆：字佐治，又稱郝參軍。晉汲郡（治所在今河南衛輝市西南）人。仕至征西參軍。⑥此過：《御覽》卷九八九作"此通"。不惡：不壞。

【釋義】

謝安起初抱有隱居東山的意願，後來朝廷徵召的命令多次下達，迫不得已，這纔就任了桓温屬下的司馬。當時有人給桓温送藥草，其中有"遠志"。桓温拿來問謝安："這種藥又叫作‘小草’，爲什麼一種藥物却有兩個名稱呢？”謝安没有馬上回答。當時郝隆在座，隨聲回答道：“這很容易解釋。待在山中就是‘遠志’，出了山林就是‘小草’。”謝安頗有慚愧之色。桓温看着謝安，笑着説：“郝參軍這句戲言並不壞，也極有意味。”

【按語】

遠志，爲多年生草本。《神農本草經》謂可“益智慧、强志”，因以功效而名之。古人認爲，此草服之可强志而致遠，故名遠志。藥用其根，稱爲“遠志”；地上部分名“小草”，亦有益精、補陰之效。古時根苗通用，現今多用“遠志”，稀用“小草”。

遠志世謂益智安神强志之品，歷代多有記述。李時珍在《本草綱目》中説：“此草服之能益智强志，故有遠志之稱。”並謂：“其功專于强志益精，治善忘。蓋精與志皆腎經之所藏也，腎經不足，則志氣衰；不能上通於心，故迷惑善忘。”早在晉代，葛洪的《抱朴子・仙藥篇》云：“陵陽子仲服遠志二十年，有子三十七人，開書所視不忘。”唐代孫思邈《千金要方》中的孔聖枕中丹，明代孫一奎《赤水玄珠》中的狀元丸，都以遠志作爲主要成分。這些方劑已被後世視爲治讀書善忘之良方，譽爲“教子弟第一方”。

“處則爲遠志，出則爲小草”雖是一句戲言，但它畢竟道出了遠志命名的一些含義，很有風趣，故流傳至今。

Milkwort Root or Thinleaf Milkwort Herb

Xie An wanted to live in seclusion originally. Later, forced by orders from the imperial court, he took the position of Si Ma[1] and became a subordinate of Huan Wen. Once a person presented some herbs to Huan Wen, among which there was Yuanzhi (milkwort root *Radix Polygalae*). Huan Wen asked Xie An, “This herb is also called ‘Xiaocao’ (*Herba Polygalae Tenuifoliae*). Why does it have two names?” Xie An did not answer. Hao Long was in presence, so he responded, saying, “This is easy to explain. While still in the mountains, it is known as ‘Yuanzhi’ (literally far-reaching aspirations). Upon leaving seclusion and entering the market, it becomes the ‘ordinary grass’.” Xie An was quite ashamed. Huan Wen looked at Xie An, laughed and said, “Officer Hao’s joke is not a bad one, and is quite illuminating."

From *A New Account of Tales of the World.*

Notes:

1. Si Ma (司馬): It was a position that existed in different Chinese dynasties, and usually functioned as the minister of war.

Editor's Note:

Yuanzhi is a perennial herb, which enhances one's brain and strengthens one's will, and hence the name. The part of Yuanzhi above the ground is called Xiaocao, with the effect of invigorating the essence and yin qi. Roots and plants were both used in the past. In nowaways, Yuanzhi is used more often, sometimes as an ingredient in formulas, while Xiaocao is seldom used. The interesting joke in the story pointed out some connotations of "Yuanzhi" and "Xiaocao," the transition between which corresponded with Xie An's life journey by that point.

【米醋療傷】

【原文】

一婢抱兒落炭火燒灼，以醋傅①之，旋愈無痕。又一少年，眼中常見一鏡②，趙卿謂之曰："來晨③以魚鱠④奉候⑤"。及期延至，從容久之，少年饑甚。見臺上一甌⑥芥醋，旋旋⑦啜⑧之。遂覺胸中豁然，眼花不見。

（選自五代 · 孫光憲《北夢瑣言》）

【注釋】

①傅：通"敷"。②一鏡：像鏡子樣的眼内翳狀物。③来晨：明天早上。④魚鱠：細切的魚肉食物。⑤奉候：恭候。⑥甌：一種盛物的小盆。⑦旋旋：隨即。⑧啜(chuò 輟) : 飲，喝。

【釋義】

有一個婢女抱着小孩，不慎將小孩子掉落在炭爐上，小孩被炭火燒傷，急用醋泥塗敷在燒傷處，傷口旋即愈合而没留下疤痕。又載：有一個少年，患眼疾，眼中常常可見一翳狀物像鏡子樣，視物昏花。醫生趙卿對他說：“明天早上，我做燒魚塊，等你來吃。”到了第二天早上，趙卿故意拖延，時間好久了，還遲遲不到。那少年饑餓已甚。他看見臺上放有一小盆芥醋，隨即把芥醋喝了。喝下去以後，馬上覺得胸中豁然，視物昏花也隨之消失了。

【按語】

《北夢瑣言》爲五代宋初孫光憲所著。作於荆州，其地古稱在雲夢以北，故據以書名。記載唐五代朝野逸聞、士大夫言行和社會風俗，其中頗多詩人軼事。

米醋，入藥多用之，因爲它含的穀物之氣很全。可消癰腫，散水氣，殺邪毒。李時珍在《本草綱目 · 穀部》第二十五卷引述《北夢瑣言》這兩則病例後說：“觀此二事，可證治癰腫，殺邪毒之驗也。大抵醋治諸瘡腫積塊，心腹疼痛，殺魚、肉、菜及諸蟲毒氣，無非取其酸收之義，而又有散瘀解毒之功。”但米醋不可多食。陶弘景說：“多食損人肌藏。”陳藏器說：“多食損筋骨，亦損胃。”望讀者慎之。

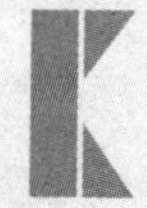

The Medical Effects of Rice Vinegar

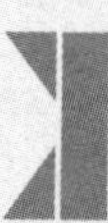

A servant girl dropped a child she was holding onto the charcoal stove, which burned the child badly. She quickly applied vinegar onto the wound, which helped the wound heal without leaving any scar. According to another record, a young man had a mirror-like nebula in eyes and could not see clearly. Doctor Zhao Qing told him, “I will cook the braised fish fillets tomorrow. Please come to eat.” In the next morning, Doctor Zhao Qing intentionally arrived late, leaving the young man starved. While waiting, the man saw a pot of mustard vinegar and drank it. After drinking the vinegar, he felt relieved in the chest and the problem of dim sight was soon gone.

From *Interesting Personalities and Anecdotes from the Tang Dynasty*[1].

Notes:

1. *Interesting Personalities and Anecdotes from the Tang Dynasty* (《北夢瑣言》Beimeng Suoyan): It is a collection of historical records in the Tang Dynasty (唐 618-907) and the Five Dynasties (五代 907-960), written by Sun Guangxian (孫光憲 901-968).

Editor's Note:

Rice vinegar is often used as medince because it contains the qi of full grain, with effects of relieving carbuncles and swelling, scattering water, killing pathogens and toxin, etc. Using too much rice vinegar may harm the liver, tendons, bones and stomach, so people should take it with caution.

【蛇銜草】

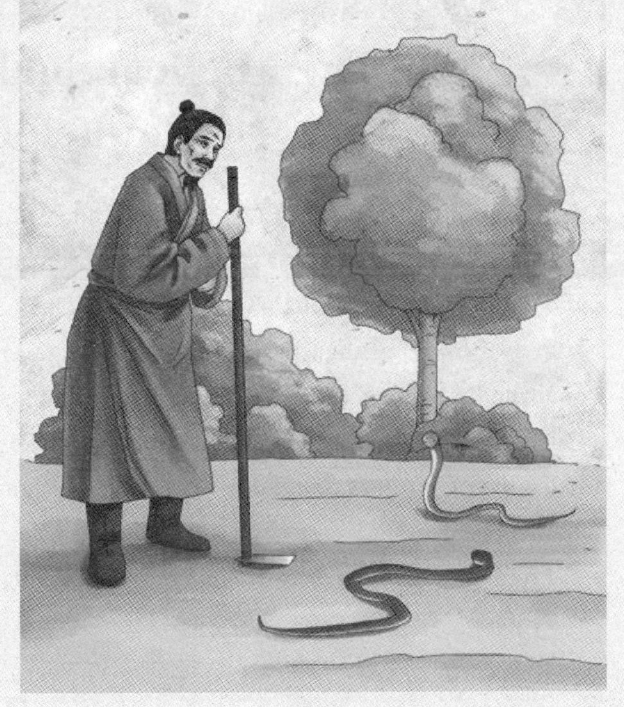

【原文】

《異苑》[①]云：昔有田父耕地，值見傷蛇在焉。有一蛇，銜草着[②]瘡上，經日傷蛇走。田父取其草餘葉[③]以治瘡，皆驗。本不知草名，因以蛇銜爲名。《抱朴子》[④]云：蛇銜能續斷之指如故是也。

（選自《太平廣記 · 草木》）

【注釋】

①異苑：志怪小説集。南朝宋劉敬叔作。十卷，記述自先秦迄劉宋的怪異之事，尤以晉代爲多。②着：附着。 ③餘葉：剩下的葉子。 ④《抱朴子》：晉 · 葛洪著。考葛洪《肘後備急方》有蛇銜膏，療癰腫、金瘡、瘀血、産後血積、耳目諸病。

【釋義】

《異苑》中記載：過去有一位老農耕地，遇見一條受了傷的蛇躺在那裏。另有一條蛇，銜來一棵草放在傷蛇的傷口上。經過一天的時間，傷蛇跑了。老農拾取那棵草其餘的葉子給人治瘡，全都靈驗。本來不知道這種草的名字，就用“蛇銜草”當草名了。《抱朴子》

說：蛇銜草能把已經斷了的手指接起來，接得和原先一樣。說的就是這回事。

【按語】

《太平廣記》是宋代李昉等人編輯的一部大型類書。因成書於宋太宗平興國年間，故名。採録自漢至宋初的小說、筆記、稗史等400多種，保存了大量的古小說资料。

蛇銜草，又稱"蛇銜""蛇含""威蛇"等。李時珍在《本草綱目》中說："其葉似龍牙而小，背紫色，故俗名小龍牙，又名紫背龍牙。"又說：該藥"主治：驚癇、寒熱邪氣、除熱、金瘡疽痔、鼠瘺惡、瘡頭瘍"等。

本文記述了蛇銜草命名的故事，於醫學頗有啓示價值。《本草綱目》將全文加以引用。而清代蒲松齡《聊齋志異》中的"鹿銜草"篇，顯然受本篇影響。

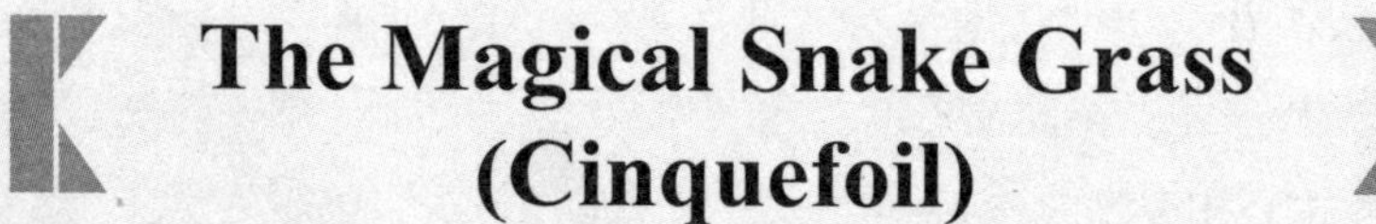

The Magical Snake Grass (Cinquefoil)

According to *Records of Odd Things*[1], there was once an old farmer cultivating the land, when he saw an injured snake lying there. Another snake took a grass in its mouth and put it onto the first snake's wound. One day later, the injured snake was healed enough to run away. Seeing this, the old farmer used the rest of grass to treat other people's wound, and proved the grass effective. He did not know the grass's name, and thus called it "Shexian Cao" (literary, the grass held in the snake's mouth). As recorded in *Book of the Master Who Embraces Simplicity* [2], this type of grass can be used in broken fingers and help them heal.

From *Extensive Records Compiled in the Taiping Years*[3].

Notes:

1. *Records of Odd Things* (《異苑》Yi Yuan): It is written by Liu Jingshu (劉敬叔) in the Former Song Dynasty (also called Liu Song Dynasty), is a supernatural fiction, which record or write about weird, uncanny or supernatural things.

2. *Book of the Master Who Embraces Simplicity* (《抱朴子》Baopuzi): Written by the Jin Dynasty scholar Ge Hong (葛洪 283-343), it is divided into esoteric *Inner Chapters* (内篇 Nei Pian) and exoteric *Outer Chapters* (外篇 Wai Pian) . *The Daoist Inner Chapters* discuss topics such as demonology, Chinese alchemy, transcending secular life, making elixirs, etc. *The Confucianist Outer Chapters* discuss Chinese literature, legalism, politics,

and so on.

3. *Extensive Records Compiled in the Taiping Years*(《太平廣記》Taiping Guangji): compiled by a famous scholar, Li Fang (李昉 925-996) , among other authors, during the Song Dynasty. It contained 500 volumes which were divided into 92 categories with different themes. It was a collection of short fictions produced from the Han Dynasty to the early Song Dynasty.

Editor's Note:

Shexian Cao is also called Shexian, Shehan, Weishe and Zibei longya. It was recorded in *Compendium of Materia Medica* written by Li Shizhen. The drug is mainly used to treat epilepsy, carbuncles, boils, and to relieve cold or heat pathogens. The excerpt provides valuable information on how the grass was named.

【苦參重腰】

【原文】

予嘗苦腰重，久坐，則旅距①十餘步然後能行。有一將佐②見予曰："得無用苦參潔齒③否？"予時以病齒用苦參數年矣。曰："此病由也，苦參入齒，其氣傷腎，能使人腰重。"後有太常少卿舒昭亮用苦參揩④齒，歲久亦病腰。自後悉不用苦參，腰疾皆愈。此皆方書舊不載者。

（選自宋 · 沈括《夢溪筆談 · 技藝》）

【注釋】

①旅距：形容走路不方便。②將佐：輔助將軍的高級軍官。③苦參：又名苦骨、地槐、水槐等。能清熱、燥濕、利水、殺蟲、止癢。潔齒：《本草綱目 · 草部 · 苦參》："《史記》云：太倉公淳于意醫齊大夫病齲齒，以苦參湯日漱三升，此亦取其去風氣濕熱、殺蟲之義。"④太常少卿：官名。掌管宗廟禮儀，少卿是太常寺的副職。揩：擦抹。

【釋義】

我曾經因腰部沉重而痛苦，久坐之後，起立走路時要艱難地慢走十幾步，然後纔能正常行走。有個將官見到我這樣，便說："你是不是用苦參潔齒了？"我當時患牙痛，用苦參擦牙已幾年了。他說："這正是引起腰痛的原因。苦參的藥氣進入牙齒。這種藥氣傷腎,會使人腰部沉重。”後來管宗廟禮儀的太常寺少卿舒昭亮用苦參擦牙,時間久了,也得了腰病。自此之後,我們都不用苦參擦牙,腰病也都好了。這些都是醫書上没有記載過的。

【按語】

《夢溪筆談》由北宋沈括所撰。因寫於潤州(治今江蘇鎮江)夢溪園而得名。分故事、辯證、樂律、象數、人事、官政、機智、藝文、書畫、技藝、器用、神奇、異事、謬誤、譏謔、雜誌和藥議十七目,凡609條。

古人以苦參漱口潔齒,實爲殺菌之意。但實踐出真知,沈括與友人舒昭亮等用之竟患腰重,發現苦參因其苦寒之性,有傷腎之弊。遂記載下來以戒後人,體現了沈括的科學態度和仁者之心。

李時珍在《本草綱目》“苦參”條下,特轉引了沈括的這段話,並説:“惟腎水弱而相火勝者,用之相宜。若火衰精冷,真元不足,及年高之人,不可用也。”清代張璐《本經逢源》亦云:“年高之人不可用也,久服苦參多致腰重。”這都證明了沈括觀點的正確和所記文獻的價值。

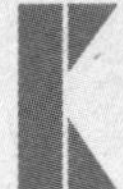

Sophora Damaging the Kidney

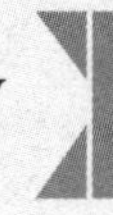

Shen Kuo recorded in *The Collection of Essays by Shen Kuo*[1] as follows: "My waist feels heavy and hurt. After sitting for a long while, I could not walk normally without walking slowly for several steps first. A general saw this and asked me whether I cleaned teeth with sophora (Kushen, Radix Sophorae Flavescentis). I admitted that I had been wiping teeth with sophora for several years due to my toothache. He then pointed out that my waist pain was due to the kidney-damaging property of sophora, which then caused burden on the waist. Later, Shu Zhaoliang, an official in charge of sacrifice and rituals, also suffered from lumber heaviness after using sophora to wipe his teeth for a long time. Since then, we stopped using it, and then the waist problem was gone. This has not been recorded in any medical book."

From *The Collection of Essays by Shen Kuo*.

Notes:

1. *The Collection of Essays by Shen Kuo* (《夢溪筆談》Mengxi Bitan): It was an

extensive book written by the Chinese polymath, scientist and statesman Shen Kuo (沈括 1031–1095) during the Song Dynasty (宋 960–1279) of China. It contains records and theories on subjects including astrology, mathematics, geology, medicine, and so on, and was a milestone in the history of science in China.

Editor's Note:

Kushen (Sophora) was used to clean the mouth and teeth because it could kill bacteria. Yet Shen Kuo and his friend found it harmful to the waist because it is bitter and cold in nature and hurts the kidney. Li Shizhen quoted this story in *Compendium of Materia Medica*, which attests to the value of this discovery and of this document.

【河豚】

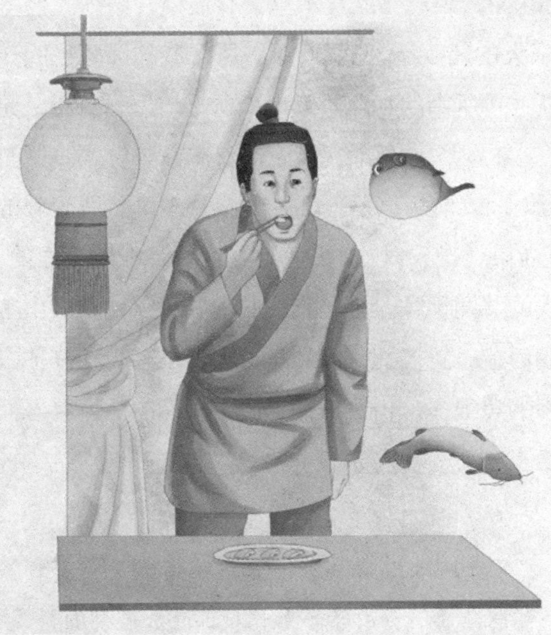

【原文】

吳人嗜河豚魚[①]，有遇毒者往往殺人，可爲深戒。據《本草》[②]"河豚味甘温，無毒，主補虛、去濕氣、理腰脚"，因《本草》有此説，人遂信以爲無毒，食之不疑，此甚誤也。《本草》所載河豚亦謂之鮠魚[③]，非人所嗜者，江浙間謂之鮰魚者是也。吳人所食河豚有毒，本名侯夷魚[④]。《本草》注引《日華子》[⑤]云河豚"有毒，以蘆根及橄欖等解之。肝有大毒。又名規魚、吹肚魚"，此乃是侯夷魚，或曰胡夷魚，非《本草》所載河豚也，引以爲注，大誤矣。規魚浙東人所呼，又有生海中者，腹上有刺，名海規；吹肚魚南人通言[⑥]之，以其腹脹如吹也。南人捕河豚法，截流爲柵，待群魚大下之時，小拔去柵，使隨流而下，日暮猥[⑦]至，自相排蹙[⑧]，或觸柵則怒而腹鼓[⑨]，浮於水上，漁人乃接取之。

（選自宋 · 沈括《夢溪筆談 · 補筆談 · 藥議》）

【注釋】

①吳人：泛指江浙一帶居民。 河豚：魨科魚類的俗稱，我國沿海均有出產，肉鮮美，但肝臟、生殖腺及血液含有毒素。②《本草》：此指宋開寶年間官修的《開寶新詳定本草》和《開寶重定本草》。 ③鮠（wéi 桅）魚：鱨科魚類，主產于長江流域，肉味鮮美，鰾可制魚肚，是上等的食用魚類。④侯夷：亦作“鯸鮐”。《本草綱目》卷四十四云：“侯夷，狀其形醜也。” ⑤《本草》注：此指宋嘉祐年間在《開寶本草》基礎上修訂成書的《嘉祐本草》之注。《日華子》：《日華子諸家本草》的簡稱，二十卷，成書於北宋開寶年間，今已佚。⑥通言：共同稱呼。 ⑦猥：衆多。⑧排蹙（cù 促）：擁擠。⑨怒而腹鼓：河豚的腹部有氣囊，遇到意外就氣囊充氣、腹部朝上浮上水面，這是河豚的一種保護性本能。古人以爲這是“怒而腹鼓”。

【釋義】

江浙一帶人嗜好河豚，有遇上中毒的往往喪命，應該深爲警惕。據《開寶本草》説“河豚味甘温，無毒，主補虚、去濕氣、理腰脚”，因爲《開寶本草》有這種説法，人們就信以爲没有毒，食用時不加懷疑，這是很大的錯誤。《開寶本草》所記載的河豚也叫作鮠魚，不是人們所嗜好的河豚，而是江浙一帶所謂的鮰魚。當地人所吃的河豚有毒，原名叫侯夷魚。《嘉祐本草》注引《日華子》説河豚“有毒，以蘆根及橄欖等解之。肝有大毒。又名規魚、吹肚魚”，這乃是侯夷魚，或稱胡夷魚，不是《開寶本草》所記載的河豚，引來作爲注解，是大謬誤。規魚是浙東一帶人对其的稱呼，還有生長在海裏面的，肚子上有刺，名叫海規；吹肚魚是南方人的共同稱呼，因爲它的肚子脹起來就像吹出來的一樣。南方人捕捉河豚魚的方法是，攔河流設置柵欄，等到魚群大批下來時稍許抽去幾根欄杆，使之順流而下，傍晚時分到來的魚很多，相互擁擠，碰上柵欄的魚就發怒而肚子鼓脹，浮在水面上，漁人便將它捕撈上來。

【按語】

本文强調河豚魚有毒，遇上中毒往往喪命，應該深爲警惕。明確指出：由於官修的《開寶本草》記載不當，使人們誤以爲河豚無毒，食用時不加懷疑，這是很大的錯誤。文中辨析了河豚的種類和不同名稱，並記載了捕捉河豚的方法。這是一篇珍貴的文獻資料。

He Tun (Fugu Fish)

People in Jiangsu and Zhejiang Provinces liked to eat He Tun (or Fugu in Japanese). It is alarming that those people often die of poisoning. According to records of *Materia Medica in Kaibao Reign*[1], He Tun is sweet in flavor and warm in nature. Non-toxic, it can tonify deficiency, remove dampness, and strengthen the waist and feet. Based on this entry, people took it as a non-toxic food and consumed it without caution. This is a big mistake. The He Tun recorded in *Materia Medica in Kaibao Reign* is also called Guiyu (Channel catfish), or Huiyu (Longsnout catfish) as the locals call it, not the favored fugu fish. Fugu taken by the local people, originally known as Houyi fish, was poisonous. According to *Material Medica in Jiayou Reign*[2], fugu is toxic, especially the liver part, which can be relieved by reed roots and olives. This is the Houyi Yu, or Huyi Yu, instead of the He Tun recorded in *Materia Medica in Kaibao Reign*. Therefore, it is a big mistake to refer to this for the property of fugu.

Guiyu is called in the eastern Zhejiang Province, while the one called Hai Gui has spikes on the abdomen and lives in the sea. Chuidu Yu (Abdomen-bulging fish) is the usual name among southern people, because their abdomens swell as they are blown out. The southern people caught fugu in such a way. First, they set up fence in the river, and then take away part of the fence to let the fish swim downward the river. By sunset, there would be plenty of fish coming and hustling each other, among which some knocked onto the fence angrily and floated on the water with swollen and expanded abdomen. The fishermen then collect the fish.

From *The Collection of Essays by Shen Kuo*.

Notes:

1. *Materia Medica in Kaibao Reign* (《開寶本草》Kaibao Bencao): Compiled by Liu Han (劉翰) and Ma Zhi (馬志) in the Tang Dynasty, it is a revision of *Newly Revised Materia Medica* (《新修本草》Xinxiu Bencao), which was compiled by Sujing (蘇敬) in the Tang Dynasty and *Materia Medica of Shu Dynasty* (《蜀本草》Shu Bencao), compiled by Han Baoyi (韓保異) in the later Shu Dynasty.

2. *Material Medica in Jiayou Reign* (《嘉祐本草》Jiayou Bencao): It is compiled by Zhang Yuxi, Linyi and Susong in Jiayou reign of the Song Dynasty (1057–1060 A. D.),

which added to the collection of herbs recorded in *Materia Medica in Kaibao Reign*.

Editor's Note:

The excerpt warns people to be careful about eating He Tun because it is toxic and may cause death. Due to the wrong information provided in *Materia Medica in Kaibao Reign*, people often thought that He Tun was non-toxic and ate it without caution. The excerpt makes an analysis about the types and different names of He Tun, and records the fishing method. This documentation is valuable as medical reference and as a piece of common knowledge.

【雞舌香】

【原文】

予集《靈苑方》①，論雞舌香以爲丁香母②，蓋出陳氏《拾遺》③，今細考之尚未然。按《齊民要術》④云：雞舌香，"世以其似丁子，故一名丁子香"，即今丁香是也。《日華子》⑤云雞舌香"治口氣"，所以三省故事⑥，郎官⑦口含雞舌香，欲其奏事對答其氣芬芳，此正謂丁香治口氣，至今方書爲然。又古方五香連翹湯用雞舌香，《千金》⑧五香連翹湯無雞舌香却有丁香，此最爲明驗。《新補本草》⑨又出丁香一條，蓋不曾深考也。今世所用雞舌香，乳香⑩中得之，大如山茱萸，銼開中如柿核，略無氣味，以治疾殊極乖謬⑪。

（選自宋・沈括《夢溪筆談・藥議》）

【注釋】

①《靈苑方》：沈括的醫學著作之一，共二十卷，今已佚，在《政和本草》中尚有該書的片斷。②丁香母：丁香系常綠喬木，其果實稱母丁香。③陳氏《拾遺》：指唐代醫學家陳藏器所編撰的《本草拾遺》。④《齊民要術》：北魏賈思勰著，十卷，是現存最早最完整的農學專著。本篇引自該書卷五中的"合香澤法"條。⑤《日華子》：見本書"河豚"條注。⑥三省：唐宋時代，中書省、門下省與尚書省並稱"三省"，是中央的主要政務機構。故事：成例。⑦郎官：泛指中央行政機構中的中級官員。⑧《千金》：指《千金方》，系唐代著名醫學家孫思邈所編撰的《備急千金要

方》與《千金翼方》兩書的統稱。 ⑨《新補本草》：即北宋嘉祐年間官修的《嘉祐補注神農本草》（簡稱《嘉祐本草》），二十卷。今已佚，其內容收入《證類本草》。⑩乳香：亦稱乳頭香，即薰陸香，產此香的樹其莖浸出的樹脂凝固後即乳香。 ⑪ 殊極乖謬：極其錯謬。乖，錯亂。

【釋義】

我纂集《靈苑方》，曾論定鷄舌香應該是母丁香，這個說法出於陳藏器的《本草拾遺》，現在仔細考究起來尚未盡然。《齊民要術》說：鷄舌香，“世人因爲它類似釘子，所以又稱它爲丁子香”，就是現在的丁香。《日華子》說鷄舌香能“治口氣”，因此三省的成例，郎官口中含鷄舌香，讓他們在陳奏事務應答時口氣芬芳，這正是所謂的丁香能治口氣，直到現在醫方書上都是這樣說的。此外，古方中的五香連翹湯用鷄舌香，《千金方》中的五香連翹湯沒有鷄舌香却有丁香，這是最爲明顯的證據。《嘉祐本草》在鷄舌香之外又列出丁香一條，是沒有深入查考。現在世上所用的鷄舌香，是從乳香中得到的，大小如同山茱萸一般，剖開來其中像柿核一樣，一點氣味都沒有，用它來治病是極其錯謬的。

【按語】

沈括曾多次論定鷄舌香就是丁香。本文針對《嘉祐本草》在鷄舌香之外又列出“丁香”一條的做法，提出批評，認爲是沒有深入查考。這是又一次對本草著作的訂正。

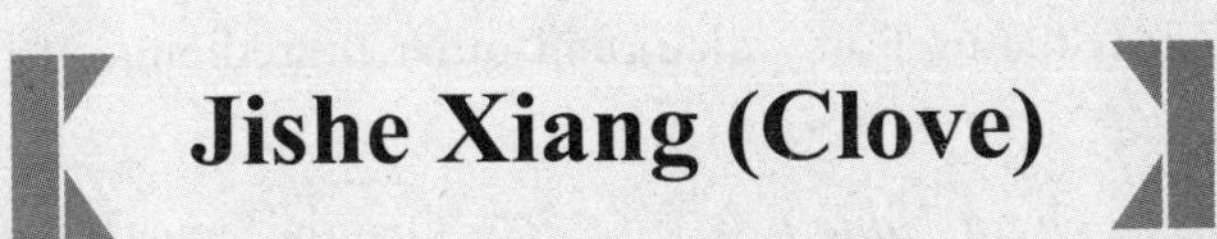

Jishe Xiang (Clove)

When I compiled *Magical Formula*[1], I thought “Jishe Xiang” refers to “Mu Dingxiang” , in accordance with *A Supplement to Materia Medica*[2] by Chen Cangqi. According to *Main Techniques for the Welfare of the People*[3], “Jishe Xiang” was also called “Dingzi Xiang” because it looks like a nail (Dingzi). That is what is currently known as cloves. According to *Materia Medica Compiled by Rihua Zi*[4], “Jishe Xiang” can refresh one’s breath. Therefore, officials are required to chew some before presenting a memorial to the emperor. That is the so-called “mouth-odor treatment” of cloves, which has been recorded in various medical books up until now. Besides, the ancient formula “Wuxiang Lianqiao Decoction[5]” used “Jishe Xiang” , while the same formula in *Prescriptions of Great Value*[6] used "Dingxiang" instead of "Jishe Xiang" . This is obvious evidence that the two were the same. "Dingxiang" also ranked besides "Jishe Xiang" in *Material Medica in Jiayou Reign* due to insufficient research and investigation. The currently used "Jishe Xiang" is made of libanus, with the same size of dogwood and no odor, looking like persimmon stone after being cut in half. It is ridiculously wrong if one to treat diseases with it.

From *The Collection of Essays by Shen Kuo*.

Notes:

1. *Magical Formula* (《靈苑方》Lingyuan Fang): It is a medical book compiled by Shen Kuo, which has been lost, though sections of it were recorded in later books.

2. *A Supplement to Materia Medica* (《本草拾遺》Bencao Shiyi): It was compiled by Chen Cangqi in the Tang Dynasty.

3. *Main Techniques for the Welfare of the People* (《齊民要術》Qimin Yaoshu): It is the most completely preserved Chinese text on agricultural techniques and practice, written by the Northern Wei Dynasty official Jia Sixie (賈思勰).

4. *Materia Medica Compiled by Rihua Zi* (《日華子》Rihua Zi): It was a medical book, compiled by Rihua Zi, an herb medicine specialist in the Tang Dynasty.

5. Wuxiang Lianqiao Decoction(五香連翹湯 Five-fragrance formula) : It is a TCM formula composed of Chenxiang (Lignum Aquilariae Resinatum), Huoxiang (Agastache rugosa), Muxiang (Radix Aucklandiae), Dingxiang (Flos Caryophylli), Shexiang (Moschus), Lianqiao (Fructus Forsythiae) and other ingredients. It has been used for treating carbuncles.

6. *Prescriptions of Great Value* (《千金方》Qianjin Fang): It is short for *Prescriptions of Great Value* for Emergencies（《備急千金要方》Beiji Qianjin Yao-fang）, sometimes the combination of *Prescriptions of Great Value* for Emergencies and *Supplement to Prescriptions of Great Value*（《千金翼方》Qianjin Yifang）. It is written by Sun Simiao, a famous traditional Chinese medicine doctor of Sui and Tang Dynasties, who was titled as "Chinese King of Medicine" (藥王 Yaowang) of China for his significant contributions to Chinese medicine.

Editor's Note:

Shen Kuo always considered "Jishe Xiang" the same as "Dingxiang" . In this excerpt, he criticized *Material Medica in Jiayou Reign* for mistakenly listing "Dingxiang" and "Jishe Xiang" as two different herbs.

【天竺黄】

【原文】

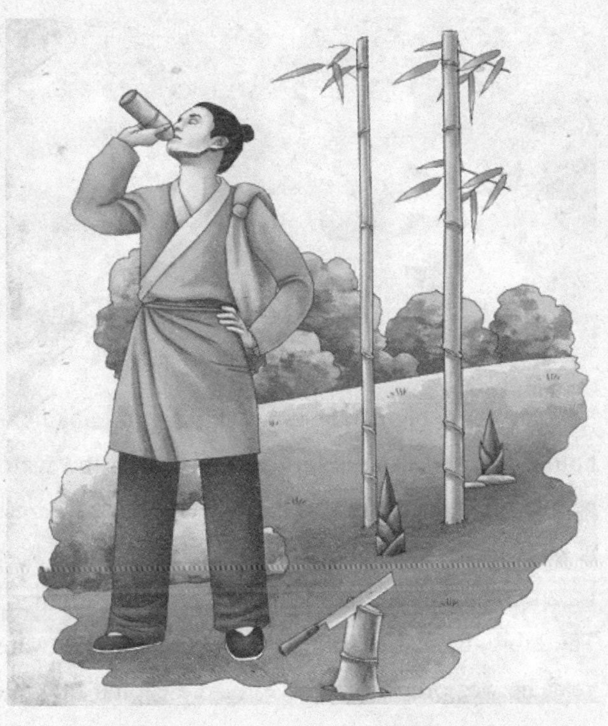

嶺南[①]深山中有大竹，有水甚清澈，溪澗中水皆有毒，唯此水無毒，土人陸行多飲之，至深冬則凝結如玉，乃天竹黄[②]也。王彥祖知雷州[③]日，盛夏之官[④]，山溪間水皆不可飲，唯剖竹取水，烹飪飲啜皆用竹水。次年被召赴闕，冬行，求竹水不可復得，問土人，乃知至冬則凝結，不復成水。遇夜野火燒林木爲煨燼，而竹黄不灰[⑤]，如火燒獸骨而輕，土人多於火後采拾以供藥，品[⑥]不若生得者爲善。

（選自宋·沈括《夢溪筆談·補筆談·藥議》）

【注釋】

①嶺南：泛指五嶺以南。 ②天竹黄：亦名竹黄，李時珍《本草綱目》卷三十七引宋僧贊寧云："竹黄生南海鏞竹中，此竹極大，又名天竹，其内有黄，可以療疾。"入藥有去風熱、治中風痰壅等功效。 ③雷州：州名，治所在今廣東海康。 ④之官：到任。之，往。 ⑤不灰：不會燒成灰。 ⑥品：品位，質地。

【釋義】

嶺南深山裏有大竹子，竹中有水相當清澈，溪澗中的水都有毒，唯獨這種水没有毒，當地人在陸地行路大多飲用它，到了隆冬竹水就凝結如玉石，這就是天竹黄。王彥祖任雷州知州時，在盛夏季節赴任，山間的溪水都不能飲用，只得剖開竹子取水，煮食、飲用都用竹子裏的水。第二年他接到命令去京城，冬天上路，找竹子裏的水却再也找不到了，詢問當地人，纔知道到冬天竹水就凝結，不再能變成水。夜間遇上野火把樹木燒成灰燼，可是竹黄不會燒成灰，如同火燒獸骨只是變輕一樣，當地人常在火燒過後采拾起來當藥用，但它的質地不如從活着的竹子中所得的好。

【按語】

本文形象地記述了天竹黄的生成、功用和制取方法，爲後人提供了珍貴的文獻資料。

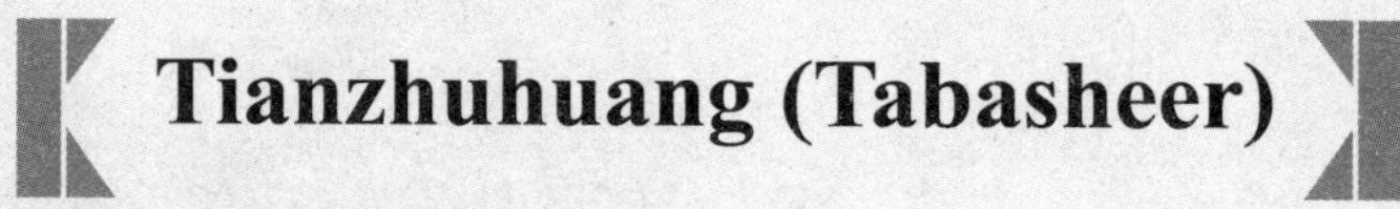

Tianzhuhuang (Tabasheer)

There are big bamboos in the deep mountains of the Lingnan region. These bamboos hold clear and drinkable water, whereas the water in the streams is toxic. The local people often drink the bamboo water, which freezes like jade in cold winter. This is what is known as Tianzhuhuang (Tabasheer). When Wang Yanzu was appointed governor of Leizhou, he passed the mountains in a midsummer, when stream water was undrinkable. Therefore, he had to split the bamboos to fetch water for drinking and cooking. The next year, he was ordered to leave for the capital in winter, when bamboo water was nowhere to find. He asked the local people and learned that the bamboo water froze in winter. In the evening, wild fire might burn the trees into ashes, not the tabasheer. They are like animal bones and would only become lighter after being burned. The local people would pick them and use them as drugs after the fire, but their quality would not be as good as the fresh ones.

From *The Collection of Essays by Shen Kuo*.

Editor's Note:

The text vividly records the formation, medical value and processing method of Tianzhu Huang, and is of great value for people of later generations.

【枳實與枳殼】

【原文】

六朝[①]以前醫方，唯有枳[②]實，無枳殼，故《本草》[③]亦只有枳實。後人用枳之小嫩者爲枳實，大者爲枳殼，主療各有所宜，遂别出枳殼一條[④]，以附枳實之後。然兩條主療，亦相出入。古人言枳實者便是枳殼，《本草》中枳實主療，便是枳殼主療。後人既别出枳殼條，便合於枳實條内摘出枳殼主療，别爲一條；舊條内只合留枳實主療。後人以《神農本經》不敢摘破，不免兩條相犯，互有出入。

（選自宋 · 沈括《夢溪筆談 · 補筆談 · 藥議》）

【注釋】

①六朝：指吴、東晉、宋、齊、梁、陳六個朝代。 ②枳(zhǐ 紙)：芸香科植物。未成熟的果實入藥稱爲枳實，成熟的稱爲枳殼。 ③《本草》：我國古來把記載藥物的著作，包括圖譜之類，稱爲本草。這裏指《神農本草經》。《神農本草經》將枳實收録於木部中品，之後，包括唐《新修本草》在内的《本草》著作都只有“枳實 ”條。④别出枳殼一條：宋初的《開寶本草》首先另立“枳殼”條。

【釋義】

六朝以前的醫方中，只有枳實而没有枳殼。所以《本草》中也只提到枳實。後人把枳的嫩小果實叫作枳實，成熟的果實叫作枳殼。因爲兩者各有不同的主要功效，于是就另列出一條枳殼，附在枳實之後。然而，這兩條的主要療效却互相有所出入。其實，古人所説的枳實就是枳殼。《本草》中所列枳實的主要功效，實際是枳殼的主要功效。後人既然另分出“枳殼”條，就應當從《本草》“枳實”條裏摘出枳殼的主要功效，另作一條，而只在舊條裏保留枳實的主要功效。後人因爲不敢打破《神農本經》的框框，不免兩條矛盾，互有出入。

【按語】

針對古代《本草》和醫方只有枳實而無枳殼的現象，沈括認真辨析了枳實與枳殼的異同和各自的功用，對《本草》著作提出了具體的修改意見。表現了認真求實的精神。這是沈括訂正《神農本經》一例。

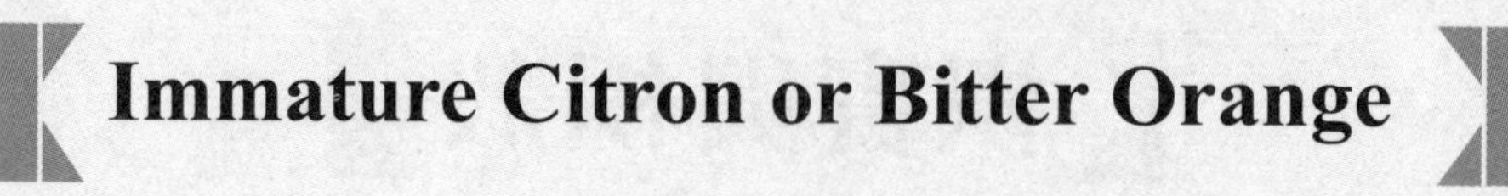

Immature Citron or Bitter Orange

There was only Zhishi and no Zhike in the medical formulas recorded before the Six Dynasties. Therefore, only Zhishi was mentioned in *King Shen Nong's Classics of Herbal Medicine* [1]. People later called the tender small citron fruits Zhishi and the ripe ones Zhike. Due to their different medicinal effects, Zhike is listed separately from Zhishi. Actually, in ancient times Zhishi was considered the same medicine as Zhike. The main curative effects of Zhishi recorded in *King Shen Nong's Classics of Herbal Medicine* were actually the main curative effects of Zhike. Now that the entry of Zhike is added, people of later generation should pick out the main curative effects of Zhike from the entry of Zhishi from *King Shen Nong's Classics of Herbal Medicine* and rank it as another entry, only keeping the main curative effects of Zhishi in the original entry. The two entries largely contradict with each other because people were afraid of violating the *King Shen Nong's Classics of Herbal Medicine*.

From *The Collection of Essays by Shen Kuo*.

Notes:

1. *King Shen Nong's Classics of Herbal Medicine* (《本草》/《神農本草經》 Bencao/ Shennong Bencao Jing): It is a Chinese book on agriculture and medicinal plants. It has been attributed to the mythical Chinese sovereign Shen Nong, who was said to have lived around 2800 BCE. Researchers maintain that this is a compilation of oral traditions written between about 300 BCE and 200. The original text no longer exists but is said to consist of three volumes with 365 entries on material medica and their description.

Editor's Note:

In ancient medical books, there were only Zhishi and no mentioning of Zhike. Shen Kuo made careful investigation and analysis of the difference, similarity and functions of Zhishi and Zhike, and his work was of great value to doctors then and after.

【野葛大毒】

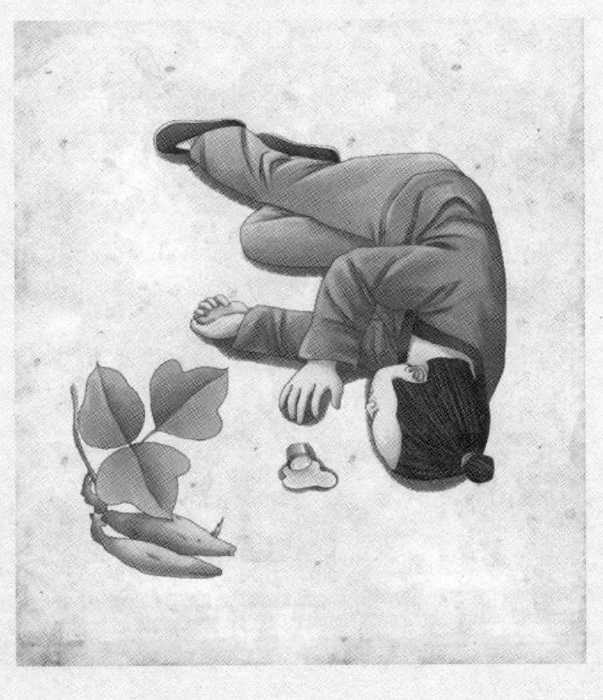

【原文】

鉤吻，《本草》[①]一名野葛，主療甚多。注釋者多端，或云可入藥用，或云有大毒食之殺人。予嘗到閩中，土人[②]以野葛毒人及自殺，或誤食者，但半葉許入口即死，以流水[③]服之毒尤速，往往投杯已卒矣。經官司勘鞫者[④]極多，灼然如此。閩人呼爲吻莽，亦謂之野葛，嶺南人謂之胡蔓，俗謂斷腸草。此草人間至毒之物，不入藥用，恐《本草》所出别是一物[⑤]，非此鉤吻也。予見《千金》《外台》[⑥]藥方中時有用野葛者，特宜仔細，不可取其名而誤用。

（選自宋・沈括《夢溪筆談・補筆談・藥議》）

【注釋】

①鉤吻：常綠纏繞灌木，屬馬錢科胡蔓藤屬，其根、莖、葉都含有劇毒。《本草》：此指《神農本草》。②土人：當地人。③流水：流動的活水。④勘鞫（jū 居）者：驗明判決的案例。如《龍門縣志》云：斷腸草“村落愚民因小忿往往嗷之以螫人”；《香山縣志》云：胡蔓草“凶民將取以毒人，……或有私怨者，茹之呷水一口則腸立斷。”宋慈《洗冤集録》中專門提到檢驗野葛中毒的症狀。⑤“别是一物”句：《神農本草》中記述的“鉤吻，一名野葛”，系馬錢科的胡蔓藤，全株均有劇毒。入藥時一般外用，有去風、攻毒、散結、消腫、止疼等作用，特别是治療疥瘡、惡瘡及跌打損傷等病有效。沈括説：“此草人間至毒之物，不入藥用，恐《本草》所出别是一物。”此結論是不準確的。實際上《本草》經中所記述的野葛和鉤吻同是一物，可入藥用。但因有劇毒，正如沈括所言：“用野葛者，特宜仔細。”另外，常用解表藥豆科中的葛根，别名也稱野葛。這種

野葛是無毒的，它與《神農本草》中記載的鉤吻之别名“野葛”，不是同科植物，屬異物同名。⑥《千金》：系唐代著名醫家孫思邈所著的《備急千金要方》與《千金翼方》兩書的統稱。《外台》：指唐代王燾所撰的《外台秘要》。

【釋義】

鉤吻，《神農本草》説又名野葛，主治的病症很多，注釋的人説法多種多樣，有的説能入藥使用，有的説有大毒吃下去會毒死。我曾到過福建，當地人用野葛來毒死他人或自殺，也有人誤吃，只要半片葉子左右入口就會死，用流動的活水送服毒性發得更快，往往剛放下杯子人已經死了，這類事經官府驗明判决的很多，其毒性就是如此顯然。福建人稱爲吻莽，也叫作野葛，嶺南人叫作胡蔓，俗稱斷腸草。這種草是世上最毒的東西，不能當藥用，恐怕《神農本草》所説的是另一種東西，不是這種鉤吻。我見到《千金方》《外台秘要》的藥方中常有使用野葛的，特别應當仔細，不能取其名稱而誤用。

【按語】

野葛即鉤吻，俗稱“斷腸草”，《吳普本草》稱“毒根”，《本草綱目》稱“爛腸草”。可見其毒性。沈括的這段記載旨在强調，野葛有大毒，稱“此草人間至毒之物”，告誡人們，用藥時“特宜仔細”，萬萬不可誤食。

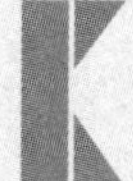

Kudzu, the Deadly Poison (Poison-ivy)

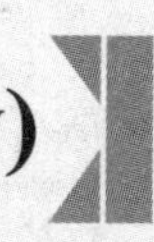

Gouwen (Conium maculatum), also called Yege in *King Shen Nong's Classics of Herbal Medicine*, differed in its property and medicinal values in different renditions. Some people said that it could be used as a drug; others thought it was poisonous, and might even cause death. I was in Fujian once, and heard of incidents of local people poisoning others or themselves with Yege, or dying of taking it by mistake. Even half a leave would kill a person. Taking with running water would increase the toxicity, causing death before one could put down the cup. There were many such cases, which were obvious evidence of its toxicity.

It is called Wen mang, or Ye ge in Fujian Province and “Hu man” or “Duanchang Cao” in the Lingnan region. It is the most toxic thing in the world, which must not be taken as drugs. I am afraid "Ye ge" recorded in *King Shen Nong's Classics of Herbal Medicine* referred to another herb, instead of "Gou wen" . "Ye ge" also appears in formulas recorded in *Prescriptions of Great Value* and *Arcane Essentials from the Imperial Library* [1]. We should be extremely cautious and should not take it by mistake.

From *The Collection of Essays by Shen Kuo*.

Note:

1. *Arcane Essentials from the Imperial Library* (《外台秘要》Waitai Miyao): It is a comprehensive medical book compiled by Wang Tao (王燾) in the Tang Dynasty.

Editor's Note:

Yege, aka Gouwen, is commonly called Duanchang Cao, or intestine-cutting grass, which indicates its toxicity. This record of Shen Kuo meant to emphasize that Yege was extremely toxic, which should be taken cautiously and not by misake.

【零陵香】

【原文】

零陵香①本名蕙，古之蘭蕙②是也，又名薰。《左傳》曰③"一薰一蕕，十年尚猶有臭"即此草也 。唐人謂之鈴鈴香，亦謂之鈴子香，謂花倒懸枝間如小鈴也。至今京師人買零陵香須擇有鈴子者。鈴子乃其花也，此本鄙語④。文士以湖南零陵郡⑤，遂附會名之。後人又收入《本草》⑥，殊不知《本草正經》⑦自有薰草條 ，又名蕙草，注釋甚明，南方處處有。《本草》附會其名，言出零陵郡，亦非也。

（選自宋 · 沈括《夢溪筆談 · 補筆談 · 藥議》）

【注釋】

①零陵香：又名佩蘭、薰草，多年生草本，屬報春花科，全草可入藥。 ②蘭蕙：《離騷》中有蘭、蕙之稱，後人以爲兩者是同一種草。 ③《左傳》曰：此處引文出自《左傳 · 僖公四年》，薰爲香草，蕕爲臭草。意謂把香草與臭草放在一起，十年之後還有臭味。 ④鄙語：指民間俗語。 ⑤零陵郡：唐代郡名，治所在今湖南零陵。 ⑥收入《本草》：五代時的《海藥本草》引陳藏器云："地名零陵，故以地爲名。"但陳氏的《本草拾遺》似未爲零陵香立條。宋初官修的《開寶本草》首先將零陵香正式收

入，亦謂其“生零陵山谷”。 ⑦《本草正經》：指《神農本草經》，但一般人們所見的乃是經陶弘景重輯的《本草經集注》。《神農本草經》中無薰草，陶弘景的《名醫别録》《本草經集注》始將其列入草部中品。沈括未加區分，就説《神農本草經》中已有“薰草”的條目了。

【釋義】

零陵香的本名叫蕙，就是古代的蘭蕙，又名叫薰，《左傳》中所説的“一薰一蕕，十年尚猶有臭”就是這種草。唐代人叫作鈴鈴香，又叫作鈴子香，指它的花倒掛在枝條中像小鈴一樣。到現在京城的人買零陵香必須挑選有鈴子的。鈴子乃是它的花，這本是民間俗語，文人因爲湖南有零陵郡，便附會爲它的名稱。後人又收進《本草》，却不知道《神農本草經》中原本就有“薰草”的條目，説它又名蕙草，注釋得很明白，南方到處都有。《開寶本草》附會它的名稱，説出産在零陵郡，也是錯誤的。

【按語】

沈括指出，零陵香本名蕙，又名薰，唐人俗語叫作鈴鈴香，南方處處有，而文人因爲湖南有零陵郡，便附會爲它的名稱。更有甚者，官修的《開寶本草》也竟然“附會其名，言出零陵郡”，這顯然是錯誤的。

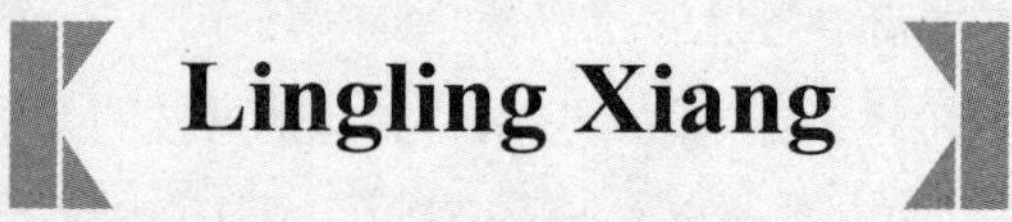

Lingling Xiang

The original name of Lingling Xiang was Hui, meaning Lanhui (Faber cymbidium; Cymbidium faberi) in the ancient times, which was also called Xun. *Chronicle of Zuo* [1] mentioned that “Xun is fragrant and You is stinky; both smells strong and long-lasting.” People in the Tang Dynasty called it Lingling Xiang, or Lingzi Xiang, as its flowers hanging inverted on the branches looked like small bells (鈴 , with the pronounciation of “ling”). Up to now, people in the capital have been picking Lingling Xiang with bell-shaped flowers. Its name also sounds like Lingling Prefecture in Hunan, and thus was also known as “Lingling” (零陵) . People of later generations kept it in records, but did not know that it was just one type of Xuncao as recorded in *King Shen Nong's Classics of Herbal Medicine*. It was also called Huicao and was everywhere in the south according to the notes. In *Materia Medica in Kaibao Reign*, the author explained its name inaccurately by attributing its origin to Lingling prefecture.

From *The Collection of Essays by Shen Kuo*.

Notes:

1. *Chronicle of Zuo* (《左傳》Zuozhuan): It is among the earliest works of narrative history in China. It is traditionally attributed to Zuo Qiuming (左丘明), a court writer of the State of Lu.

Editor's Note:

Shen Kuo pointed out that Lingling Xiang (零陵香)was also called Hui, Xun, or Lingling Xiang (鈴鈴香). It was named after Lingling prefecture of ancient Hunan because it was so common in the south. But *Materia Medica in Kaibao Reign* recorded Lingling prefecture as its origin, which was an obvious mistake.

李防禦治痰嗽

【原文】

李防禦①，京師人。初爲入内醫官，直嬪御閣②妃苦痰嗽，終夕不寐，面浮如盤。時方有甚寵，徽宗幸其閣③，見之以爲慮，馳遣呼李。李先用數藥，詔令往内東門供狀：若三日不效當誅。

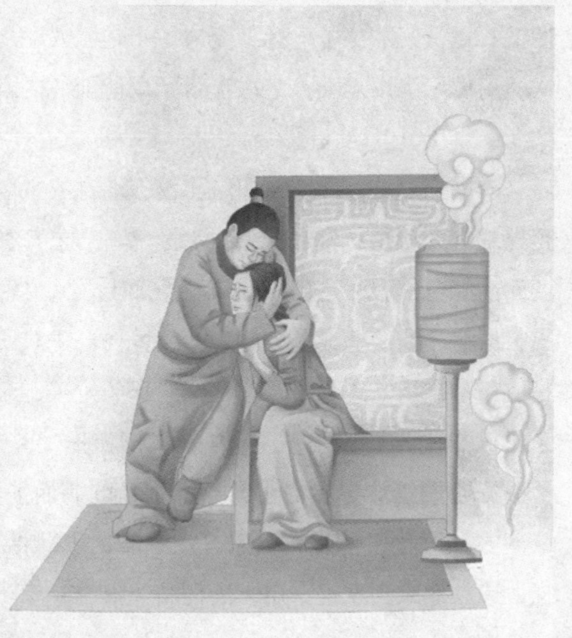

李憂撓技窮，與妻對泣。忽聞外間叫云："咳嗽藥一文一貼。吃了今夜得睡。"李使人市④藥十貼，其色淺碧，用淡虀水⑤滴麻油數點調服。李疑草藥性獷，或使藏府滑泄，並三爲一。自試之。既而無他。于是取三貼合爲一，攜入禁庭，授妃。請分兩服以餌。是夕嗽止，比[⑥]曉面腫亦消。內侍走白[⑦]，天顏絶喜[⑧]。錫[⑨]金帛，厥直萬緡[⑩]。

李雖幸其安，而念必宣索方書，何辭以對？殆[⑪]亦死爾。命僕俟[⑫]前賣藥人過，邀入坐，飲以巨鍾。語之曰："我見鄰里服汝藥多效，意欲得方，倘以傳我，此諸物爲銀百兩，皆以相贈不吝。"曰："一文藥安得其值如此？防禦要得方，當便奉告。只蚌粉一物，新瓦炒令通紅，拌青黛少許爾。"扣其所從來[⑬]，曰："壯而從軍，老而停汰[⑭]，頃見主帥有此，故剽得之。以其易辦，姑藉以度餘生，無他長也。"

（選自宋・張杲《醫説・治痰嗽》）

【注釋】

①防禦：職官名。②直嬪御閣："直"同"值"，遇到。嬪御閣：皇帝的嬪妃的住處。③其閣：指皇帝這位愛妃住的嬪御閣。④市：買。⑤虀（jī 機）水：醃菜水。虀：切碎的醃菜。⑥比：及，等到。⑦走白：跑來告説。⑧天顏：皇上。絶喜：很高兴。⑨錫：通"賜"。⑩厥直：其值。直，同"值"，價值。緡：成串的錢，一千文爲一緡。⑪殆：表示揣测的語氣。⑫俟：等待。⑬扣：問。所從來：從哪裏得來。⑭停汰：指停餉淘汰。

【釋義】

李防禦是開封人。當初他做宮廷裏的醫官時，正值嬪御閣的一位妃子患痰嗽病，整夜不能安寐，臉腫得像盤子一樣。當時這個妃子很受宋徽宗的寵愛。徽宗皇帝來到嬪御閣，看見愛妃的樣子，感到憂慮，于是派人馳馬叫李防禦來診治。因爲李防禦先前曾數次給這位妃子用過藥，這次皇帝詔令他前往内宮東門立下狀書，如果三天内治不好妃子的病，當伏誅。

李防禦爲自己的醫術用盡而憂慮苦惱，抓撓不安，與妻子相對哭泣。這時忽然聽到外邊有人叫道："咳嗽藥一文錢一劑，吃了今夜就能安睡。"李防禦派人買了十劑藥，藥面淺緑色，服法是用淡醃鹹菜湯加上幾滴麻油調服。李防禦恐怕草藥性烈，吃下後使臟腑滑泄，他便把藥並三劑爲一劑，自己先試服。服藥後，也没發現什麼不舒之處。于是取三劑合爲一劑，帶入宮廷交給那位妃子，請她分兩次服用。當晚病人咳嗽停止，等到次日清晨臉腫也消退了。内侍跑來稟報，皇上很高興，賞賜金帛，其價值萬緡。

李防禦雖然慶幸自己因治愈妃子的病而能平安無事，但又想到皇上必然要向他索取藥方，那該用什麼話來回答呢？恐怕也難活命。于是命僕人在門前等候那賣藥人經過，邀請他來到家裏，用大酒杯請他喝酒。李防禦對他説：我看見鄰居們服了你的藥大多有效，我想得到這個藥方，倘若能把它傳給我，這些東西值一百兩銀子，我全部送給你，毫不吝惜。”那賣藥的人說：“一文錢的藥怎麼能值這麼些錢呢？防禦想要得到此方，我便告訴您。只需蚌粉一物，在新瓦上炒得通紅，拌上一點青黛就行了。”李防禦又問這個藥方從哪裏得來，賣藥人答道：“我壯年時當兵，年老被停餉淘汰，一個偶然機會，我見主帥有這個藥方，就把它偷到手。因爲這種藥容易制作，姑且借賣藥來度我的餘年，此外我就没其他本事了。”

【按語】

張杲把南宋以前的文史著作和其他雜著中有關醫學典故及傳説整理成書，取名《醫説》。

這則故事，曾廣爲流傳。清代名醫趙學敏在《串雅序》中說：“李防禦治嗽得官，傳方於下走。誰謂小道不有可觀者歟？”指的就是這件事。“下走”指的是民間的走方醫。御醫李防禦，在走投無路、萬般無奈之際，向民間的走方醫求得單方，治愈了宋徽宗愛妃的痰嗽病，也保住了自己的性命，並升了官。這一事實告誡人們：不可輕視民間驗方，單方往往能治大病。在那些走街串巷的走方醫中，在廣大的民間百姓中，蘊藏着許多有價值的驗方，這是祖國醫學寶庫中不可或缺的一部分，應當認真去發掘。

Li Fangyu Treated Cough with Phlegm

Li Fangyu lived in the capital Bianliang. When he was a medical official in the royal court, an imperial concubine coughed with phlegm. She could not sleep well and her face swelled really badly. Emperor Huizong of Song favored her and was worried after visiting her, so he called for Li Fangyu to examine her. Since Li Fangyu had treated her several times, the emperor ordered him to sign a written oath at the eastern gate of the inner palace, saying that he would be executed if he still could not cure her.

Having no idea how to proceed this time, Li Fangyu felt anxious and cried together with his wife. It was right then when he heard a person shouting outside, “Cough drugs, one Wen[1] one dose. Take it and sleep well!” Li Fangyu sent people to get ten doses of the drug, which was light green, powdered and to be taken with pickle paste and several drops of sesame oil. Li Fangyu was unsure of the potency and property of the drug, and afraid that it might cause loose bowels and diarrhea. Therefore, he combined three doses of drugs and took it for a try. He did not feel any discomfort after taking it, and presented one big dose of the drug to the concubine. The patient stopped coughing the very evening, and her face no longer swollen the next morning. The royal servants passed on the news to the emperor, who was greatly delighted. Li was awarded with gold and silk.

Li Fangyu felt rejoiced for having cured the concubine, but he was still worried about a potential inquiry from the emperor about the formula. Therefore, he managed to find the drug seller and invited him for generous servings of wine. Li Fangyu told him, "Your drug proved to be quite effective, and I would like to know the formula. If you could tell me, I will send you a hundred taels of silver." The drug seller said, "How could the one-Wen drug be so valuable? If you do want to know, I will tell you. You just need to stir-bake the oyster powder on a new tile until it becomes bright red, and then mix it with Qingdai." Li then asked him where he got the formula. The man answered, "I joined the army when I was young and was cast out after I became old. I accidentally saw the formula in the general's room and stole it. The drug is easy to make and can support me for the rest of my life. I have no other means to make a living now."

From *on Medicine*.

Notes:

1. Wen (文): It is a former monetary unit, equal to 1/1000 tael of silver.

Editor's Note:

This excerpt has been well known. The imperial doctor Li Fangyu found a formula from a folk doctor to cure the bad cough of the emperor's concubine. As a result, he saved his life and was promoted. People should learn from this story the value of folk formulas. A single, inexpensive formula might cure a tricky disease. Many ordinary people and unknown doctors on the street held valuable formulas. These formulas are also an integral part of TCM, and deserved study and respect.

【車前止暴下】

【原文】

歐陽文忠公①嘗得暴下，國醫不能愈。夫人云："市人②有此藥，三文一貼，甚效。"公曰："吾輩藏府與市人不同，不可服。"夫人便以國醫藥雜進③之，一服而愈。召賣藥者，厚遺④之。求其方，乃肯傳。但用車前子一味爲末，米飲下二錢匕。云："此藥利水道而不動氣，水道利則清濁分，穀臟⑤自止矣。"

（宋・張杲《醫説・車前止暴下》）

【注釋】

①歐陽文忠公：即歐陽修，"文忠"是他的謚號。②市人：走街串巷治病賣藥的走方醫。③雜：雜和，摻和。進：服用。④遺（wèi 畏）：饋贈。⑤穀臟：腸胃。此指代腸胃的水瀉病。

【釋義】

歐陽修曾患急性水瀉，國醫不能治愈。他夫人說："街市上的走方醫有治此病的藥，三文錢一貼，很有效驗。"歐陽修說"：我們這些人的臟腑跟一般人不同，不能服用他們的藥。"夫人不便多言，便在國醫的藥中悄悄地摻和了走方醫的藥給丈夫服用，一服病竟然好了。事後歐陽修叫來賣藥的人，用厚禮酬謝他，向他索取醫方，那人才肯傳授。原來只是用一味車前子研成細末，用米湯送服二錢匕左右。那人說："此藥通利水道但又不擾動正氣，水道通利，大小便就正常，這樣腸胃病自然就好了。"

【按語】

這一事例同"李防禦治痰嗽"一樣，都是説明民間走方醫的治方頗有可取之處。清代名醫趙學敏在《串雅序》中説："昔歐陽子暴利幾絶，乞藥於牛醫。"指的就是此事。那些"乘華軒、繁徒衛"的國醫們，往往瞧不起走街串巷的走方醫，甚至污稱他們爲"牛醫"，而正是這位被稱作"牛醫"的民間醫生，在衆多御醫束手無策的情況下，竟治愈了朝廷重臣的危疾，使幾乎絶命的歐陽修轉危爲安。豈不發人深思。

Plantain Stopped Diarrhea

Once Ouyang Xiu suffered from acute diarrhea, which even the renowned masters could not cure. His wife said, “The wandering practitioners on the street have a cheap and effective formula for this disease.” Ouyang Xiu answered, “We have different internal organs with ordinary people, and therefore we cannot take the same drug.” His wife could not persuade him, so she mixed the cheap drug with that prescribed by imperial physicians. After taking the mixed drugs, Ouyang Xiu recovered unexpectedly. Later, Ouyang Xiu invited the wandering drug-seller to reward him. The man then agreed to tell him the composition of the formula: grind Cheqian Zi and take it with rice soup. He said that the drug cleansed the water passage without disturbing the vital qi. Keeping a smooth water passage and normal excrement and urination would naturally cure a problem with the intestines and stomach.

From *on Medicine*.

Editor’s Note:

This excerpt also shows the value of folk medicine, which was often looked down upon by doctors with official titles. Folk doctors were even called “cattle doctors.” However, in this story folk medicine saved the great minister Ouyang Xiu when imperial doctors could not help.

芋梗解蜂毒

【原文】

處士[1]劉易，隱居王屋山[2]。嘗於齋中見一大蜂罹[3]於蜘蛛網，蛛搏之，爲蜂螫墜地。俄頃，蛛鼓腹[4]欲裂，徐徐行入草，蛛齧[5]芋梗微破，以瘡就齧處摩之，良久，腹漸消，輕捷如故。自後人有爲蜂螫者挼[6]芋梗敷之，即愈。

（選自宋 · 彭乘[7]《續墨客揮犀》）

【注釋】

①處士：舊時讀書人，不願爲官而隱居者稱處士。 ②王屋山：在山西省垣曲、河

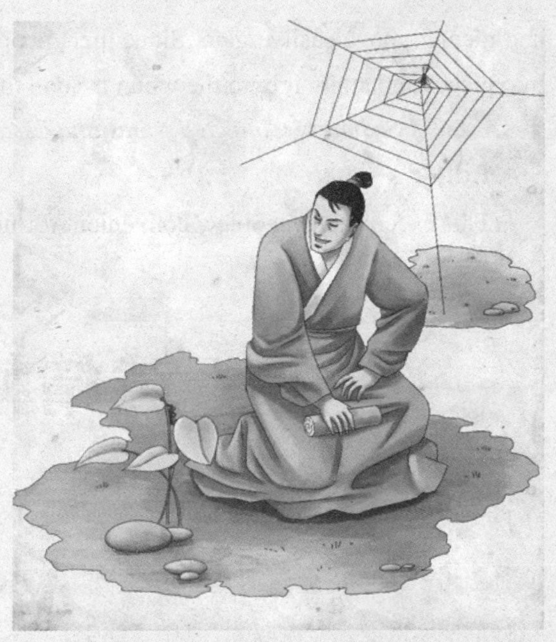

南省濟源等之間，是中條山的支脈，濟水發源地。 ③罹（lí離）：遭遇不幸。 ④鼓腹：指腹脹如鼓。 ⑤齧(niè聶)：咬。 ⑥挼(ruó)：揉搓。 ⑦彭乘：北宋學者。字利建，益州華陽（今四川成都）人，生卒年皆不詳，約宋哲宗年間人。著有《墨客揮犀》《續墨客揮犀》各十卷。内容爲宋代遺聞軼事，以及詩話文評，徵引頗爲詳洽。《續墨客揮犀》是宋人筆記中罕傳之書。自明代萬曆年間商浚刻入《稗海》中，始爲流傳。

【釋義】

劉易是位讀書人，不願做官，隱居在王屋山中。有一次他在書房裏見一隻大蜂碰在蜘蛛網上，蜘蛛與蜂搏鬥，被蜂螫傷掉在地上。不一會，蜘蛛腹部鼓起像要裂開一樣，它慢慢地爬入草叢中，用嘴咬破芋頭梗，以蜂螫處摩擦好久，腹脹消退，輕捷如常。自此之後，凡人被蜂螫的，就把芋頭秧子揉碎敷於患處，即可痊愈。

【按語】

這則故事告知人們一個便驗良方，即芋梗解蜂毒。唐《大明本草》云："芋梗，擦蜂毒尤良。"宋·寇宗奭《本草衍義》云："塗蜘蛛傷。"故此方值得推廣。

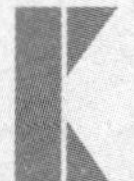

Taro Stem for Relieving Wasp Sting

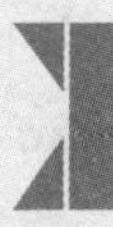

Liu Yi was a scholar. He did not want to be an official and lived in seclusion in the Wangwu Mountain. Once he saw a big wasp flying onto spider's web. The spider fought with the wasp, was stung by it and fell onto the ground. Soon, the spider's abdomen swelled like it was going to break. It slowly crawled into the grass, bit the taro stem, and rubbed the wound with the stem for a long time. Then its abdominal swell was reduced and it could move easily again. Since then, people stung by wasps would break taro stems into pieces and apply it onto the wound. Soon they will recover.

From *A Sequal to Collected Notes and Essays by Peng Cheng*.

Editor's Note:

This excerpt tells people a convenient formula, and how it was discovered.

【黄精輕體】

【原文】

臨川① 有士人,虐②,遇其所使婢,婢不堪其毒,乃逃入山中。久之,糧盡饑甚,坐水邊,見野草枝葉可愛，即拔取濯③水中，連根食之甚美。自是恒食，久之遂不饑，而更輕健。夜息大樹下，聞草中獸走以爲虎而濯，因念得上樹杪④，乃佳也；正爾念之，而身已在樹杪矣。及曉，又念當下平地，又歘然⑤ 而下。自是意有所之⑥，身輒⑦ 飄然而去，或自一峰之一峰頂，若飛鳥焉。數歲，其家人伐薪見之，以告其主，使捕之不得。一日遇其在絶壁下，即以網三面圍之，俄而騰上山頂，其主益駭異，必欲致之。或曰：此婢也，安有仙骨？不過得靈藥餌之爾。試以盛饌⑧ ，多具五味，令甚香美，置之往來之路，觀其食之否。如其言，果來就食，食訖，不復能遠去，遂爲所擒，具述其故。問其所食草之形，即黄精也。

（選自宋 · 徐鉉《稽神録》⑨）

【注釋】

① 臨川：今江西臨川縣西。 ②虐：殘暴狠毒。 ③ 濯（zhuó，酌）：洗。④ 杪（miǎo 秒）：樹梢。⑤歘（chuà）然：形容走起路來整齊的脚步聲。 ⑥之：往，到。 ⑦ 輒：總是。 ⑧饌（zhuàn 篆）：飯食。 ⑨《稽神録》：北宋文人徐鉉撰《稽神録》，六卷，是一部志怪小説集。記述唐末五代異聞，多爲靈異神怪之事。雖有荒誕不經之處，但有些資料仍有參考價值。其中故事，大都收入《太平廣記》。

【釋義】

過去江西臨川縣有個官人，對他的奴婢十分殘暴兇狠，説打就打，説駡就駡，有一個女傭人實在忍受不了，于是就逃進深山野林裏。時間長了，所帶的糧食已經吃完，肚子已經空了，非常饑餓，坐在水溝邊，看見一棵野草的枝葉長得十分可愛，就拔了一棵在水裏洗了洗，連根帶葉吃了些，味道還很好。從此就常以這種植物爲食物來充饑，時間長了就没有饑餓感了，反而行動輕便矯健。晚上到大樹下睡覺，聽到草叢中有走獸跑動，自以爲是老虎來洗澡而恐懼害怕，心裏想上樹梢最保險，正想之間這時身體已經到了樹梢。等到天剛亮的時候，心裏剛有下樹的意念，身子隨着欻欻的脚走聲，就已經到了樹下。只要意念想到哪裏，她就非常輕鬆地像飛到哪裏一樣，有時從這一峰頂到那一峰頂，行動像飛鳥般的輕快。時間一晃已過了數年。那個殘酷兇狠的舊主人家裏，有人上山砍柴偶爾發現了這個女奴婢，回家後告訴了他的主人，然後派人逮她，也没有捕捉到。有一天正碰上她在懸崖絶壁下面，立即用網三面圍住她，突然間她騰空而起，躍上了山頂。她的主人更覺得驚奇了，就越想逮住她。有的人說："這個女婢，哪裏有仙骨呢？大概是在深山中吃了神藥吧。"爲了逮住她，就設法在她來往的路上，放着五味俱全、十分香美的食物做誘餌，來觀察她到底吃不吃。果然不出所料，她看見了豐盛的食物就吃，吃完了以後，就跑得不快了，于是就被逮住了，然後她詳細講述了這其中的緣故。問後才知道她吃的那種植物，就是黄精。

【按語】

關於黄精的這個傳説，在宋代唐慎微的《證類本草》和明代李時珍的《本草綱目》中，均有引用。雖然有些神奇的色彩，但黄精的輕身健體之功，不可埋没。梁代陶弘景《名醫别録》云：黄精"氣味甘平無毒。主治補中益氣，除風濕，安五臟。久服輕身延年不饑"。李時珍在《本草綱目》中説："黄精爲服食要藥，故《名醫别録》列於草部之首，仙家以爲芝草之類，以其得坤土之精粹，故謂之黄精。"可見黄精確是一味補益之品。

Huang Jing (Solomonseal) Lightens Human Body

Once there were an official in Linchuan County of Jiangxi Province. He was bad-tempered and cruel to his servants, beating and scolding them at will. A maid couldn't bear him, and thus ran to hide in the mountain forest. In a few days, she ate up all the food she brought and felt really hungry. Sitting beside a ditch, she found a fine-looking grass, and picked its leaves to eat. The plant filled her up and made her strong, vigorous and agile. In the evening, she slept under a big tree. Hearing some sounds from the beasts in the grass, she was worried and thought about how nice it would be to stay on the top of the tree. With this thought, she quickly climbed onto the tree. At dawn, with the intention of going down, she quickly went under the tree. From then on, she could easily go everywhere she wanted, from one mountaintop to another, brisk like a bird. After several years, someone went to the mountain for firewood and ran into her. The man returned to tell her former master. The master then sent people to catch her but failed. One day when she was standing under a cliff, the master ordered his servants to besiege her from all directions. Suddenly she jumped upward onto the mountaintop, which shocked the master and made him more eager to catch her. Some people said, "How could such a servant become so extraordinary? Perhaps she had eaten some magical drugs in the deep mountain." In order to catch her, the master had delicious food served on the road she passed as baits. As expected, she took the delicious food and could not run fast any more. When being caught, she explained the reason to others and the plant she ate was identified as Huangjing.

From *Deities, Spirits and Immortals*.

Editor's Note:

Though the excerpt was exaggerating, the effects of Huangjjng should not be denied. Huangjing is a tonic drug, sweet in flavor and mild in property. It can enrich the essential qi, relieve rheumatism, and soothe the five organs. After taking it for a long time, one becomes more vigorous and one's life span prolonged.

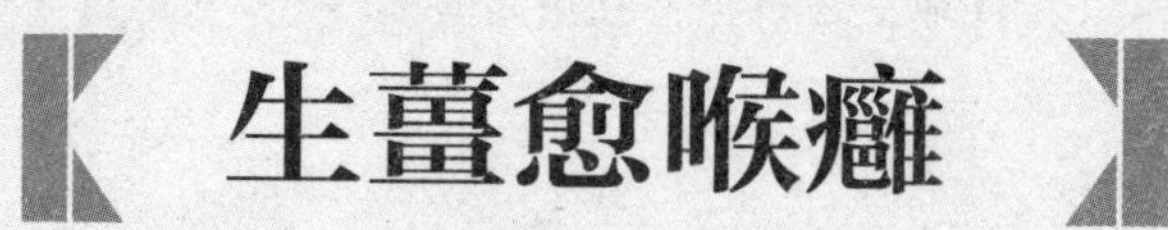

生薑愈喉癰

【原文】

楊立之自廣州府通判歸楚州①，喉間生癰，既腫潰而膿血流注，曉夜不止，寢食俱廢，醫者爲之束手。適楊吉老②來赴，郡守③招立之兩子走往邀之，至，熟視④良久曰："不許看脈，已得之矣。此疾甚異，須先啗⑤生薑片一斤，乃可投藥。否則，無法也。"語畢即去。子有難色，曰："喉中潰膿痛苦，豈宜食薑？"立之曰："吉老醫術通神，其言

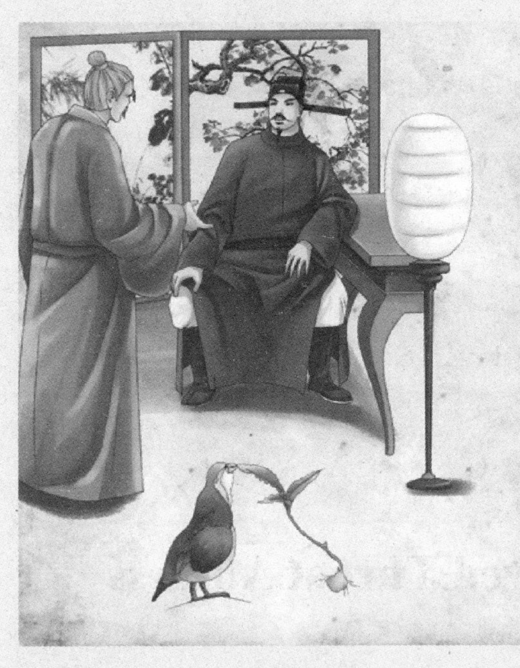

必不妄。試以一二片啗我，如不能進，則屏去[⑥]無害。”遂食之。初時殊[⑦]爲甘香，稍[⑧]復加益，至半斤許痛處漸已；滿一斤始覺味辛辣，膿血頓盡，粥餌入口無滯礙。明日招吉老謝而問之，對曰：“君官南方，必多食鷓鴣[⑨]，此禽好嚼半夏，久而毒發，故以薑制之。今病源已清，無用服他藥也。”

（選自宋 · 洪邁[⑩]《夷堅志》）

【注釋】

①通判：宋置官名。地位略次於州府長官，號稱監州。楚州：今江蘇省淮河以南，盱眙以東，鹽城以北地區。 ②楊吉老：名介，北宋泗州（今安徽省盱眙）人。崇寧間（1102—1106），郡守李夷行命令醫生、畫工剖視繪圖。楊吉老曾剖腹觀察繪製《存真圖》一卷，今佚。 ③郡守：地方行政長官，即太守。 ④熟視：仔細觀察。 ⑤啗（dàn 淡）：“啖”的異體字。 ⑥屏去：除去。 ⑦殊：很。 ⑧稍：逐漸。 ⑨鷓鴣：鳥名。多食半夏苗、植物種子和昆蟲之類。肉鮮味美，可供食用。 ⑩洪邁：見《張鋭起死回生》一文注釋。

【釋義】

楊立之從廣州府的通判任上返回楚州，咽喉生癰瘡紅腫，潰破膿血流出如注，晝夜不停，飲食不進，夜不能眠，衆醫束手無策。正遇楊吉老先生到楚州來，楚州郡守便招呼楊立之的兩個兒子速往邀請楊吉老來診治，吉老來到，仔細觀察了好大一會兒説：“不必診脈，已經曉得致病原因了。這病很特殊，必須先吃生薑一斤，然後才能服藥。若不這樣，就無法治療。”説罷他就走了。楊立之的兒子臉有難色，很不高興地説：“咽喉潰膿疼痛難忍，怎麼能適合吃生薑呢？”楊立之説：“吉老先生醫術神妙，他絶對不説謊話，先給我一兩片生薑試試看，如果不能吃下，再擯棄不用也没害處。”于是就吃生薑。剛一吃就感覺薑的味道非常甘甜而香，逐漸再增加量，吃到半斤時，咽喉疼痛漸漸消失；吃够生薑一斤，開始感覺薑味辛辣，膿血停止，米粥入口亦覺通暢。到了第二天，把楊吉老請來道謝，並詢問其中的原因。楊吉老對楊立之説：“你在南方做官，必然多吃鷓鴣，此鳥好吃半夏，時間長了，半夏之毒侵及咽喉，故導致喉癰潰流膿血不止。生薑專解半夏之毒，所以讓你先吃生薑一斤而制之。現在致病因素已經清除，不必再吃別的藥了。”

【按語】

《夷堅志》由南宋洪邁撰。原有四百二十卷。已殘闕。

這則故事，介紹了生薑解半夏之毒而治愈喉癰的功效，同時從中可以看出楊吉老的豐富閱歷和高超醫術。李時珍在《本草綱目・禽部・鷓鴣》中也引用了這則故事，以說明多食鷓鴣亦有毒。正是因爲生薑能解半夏之毒，所以後來人們多用薑汁炮製半夏，以便更好地發揮藥效。

Fresh Ginger Dissolved Throat Abscess

When Yang Lizhi returned to Chuzhou from his official appointment in Guangzhou prefecture, he suffered from a throat carbuncle, sore and swelling. Pus and blood continuously flowed out due to the diabrosis, making him unable to eat or sleep. Many doctors were called for but failed to cure him. Since the old doctor Yang Jilao happened to be Chuzhou then, the governor of Chuzhou sent for Yang Jilao. Doctor Yang carefully examined Lizhi for a while and said, “pulse-taking is not necessary as I can see the cause of the problem. Your conditions are unique, and you need to eat half a kilogram of fresh ginger before taking drugs. If not, the disease is incurable.” Then he left. Reluctant and displeased, Yang Lizhi’s son said, “How could my father eat fresh ginger with such pain and sore throat?” Yang Lizhi said, “Doctor Yang was highly regarded and wouldn’t prescribe ginger for no good reason. Let me try to eat one or two slices of fresh ginger. It has no harm to have a try.” Then he took the fresh ginger. At first, the ginger tasted sweet and fragrant so he took more. After taking half a quarter of a kilogram, his throat pain gradually disappeared. After taking half a kilogram, the pus and blood stopped flowing out. The ginger started to taste pungent to him as to a healthy person, and now the rice porridge was easy to swallow. The next day, he invited Doctor Yang to thank him and to make an inquiry. Yang Jilao told Lizhi, “As an official in the south, you’ve certainly eaten many partridges. The bird loves eating Banxia, thus the poison of Banxia gradually invaded the throat, causing the throat abscess, pus and blood. Fresh ginger can relieve the poison of Banxia, thus I asked you to take fresh ginger. Now that the pathogenic cause has been figured out and the problem solved, you don't have to take any drugs."

From *A Collection of Hearsay and Anecdotes*.

Editor's Note:

The excerpt reveals that fresh ginger can dissolve Banxia's toxin and cure throat carbuncles. It also shows the rich experiences and proficient medical skills of Yang Jilao. Since fresh ginger can relieve Banxia's toxin, people often prepare Banxia with ginger juice to maximize its effects and minimize its harm.

【覆盆子葉除眼疾】

【原文】

潭州趙太尉母病爛弦疳眼二十年。有老嫗云："此中有蟲，吾當除之。"入山取草蔓葉，咀嚼，留汁入筒中。還以皂①紗蒙眼，滴汁漬②下弦。轉盼間蟲從紗上出，數日下弦乾。復如法滴上弦，又得蟲數十而愈。後以治人多驗，乃覆盆子葉也，蓋治眼妙品。

（選自宋 · 洪邁《夷堅志》）

【注釋】

①皂：黑色。 ②漬：浸潤。

【釋義】

潭州趙太尉的母親患爛眼瞼病二十年。有一老太婆說："眼中有蟲，我可以把它除掉。"她就進山采了一些蔓草的葉子，在口中咀嚼，然後把汁擠入竹筒中。再用黑紗把病人的眼蒙上，把葉汁滴在黑紗上，以浸漬下眼瞼。轉眼工夫，蟲就從黑紗上鑽出，後來用此法滴上眼瞼，又出來數十隻蟲子，數日後下眼瞼痊愈。後來用此法治這種眼病的大都很應驗，這就是覆盆子葉，它是治眼病的奇效藥品。

【按語】

李時珍在《本草綱目 · 草部》"覆盆子"條下引述了洪邁的這段記載。他在論述覆盆子葉的功能時説："挼絞取汁，滴目中，去膚赤，出蟲如絲線。明目止淚。"除了用其葉治眼疾外，臨床多用其子。陶弘景《名醫別録》云："名覆盆，以其形圓而扁，如釜如盆，就蒂結倒垂向下，一如盆之下覆也。"因稱覆盆子。臨床上借覆盆子益腎、固精、縮尿的功能，來治療腎虛不固的遺精、遺尿，以及陽痿不育、目暗不明等證。

Raspberry Leaves Cured Eye Diseases

The mother of Zhao Taiwei in Tanzhou had rotten eyelid for twenty years. An old woman said to her, "There are insects in your eyes. I can get rid of them." Then she went into the mountain, picked some raspberry leaves, chewed them and squeezed the juice into a bamboo tube. She covered the patient's eyes with a piece of black cotton gauze, dropped the juice onto the gauze to cover the lower eyelid. Soon the insects crawled out from the black gauze, and several days later the lower eyelid recovered. It was effective in treating many people's eye diseases.

From *A Collection of Hearsay and Anecdotes*.

Editor's Note:

According to the record in *Compendium of Materia Medica*, raspberry leaves and seeds can be used to cure eye diseases. With effects of nourishing the kidney, consolidating the essence and constraining the urine, raspberry is also clinically used to treat seminal emission, enuresis, impotence, and infertility.

【白及補肺】

【原文】

台州獄吏憫[①]一大囚。囚感之，因言：“吾七次犯死罪，遭拷訊，肺皆損傷，至於嘔血。人傳一方，只用白及爲末，米飲日服，其效如神。”後其囚凌遲[②]，劊者割其胸，見肺間竅穴數十處，皆白及填補，色猶不變也。洪貫之聞其説，赴任洋州[③]，一卒忽苦咯血甚危，用此救之，一日即止也。

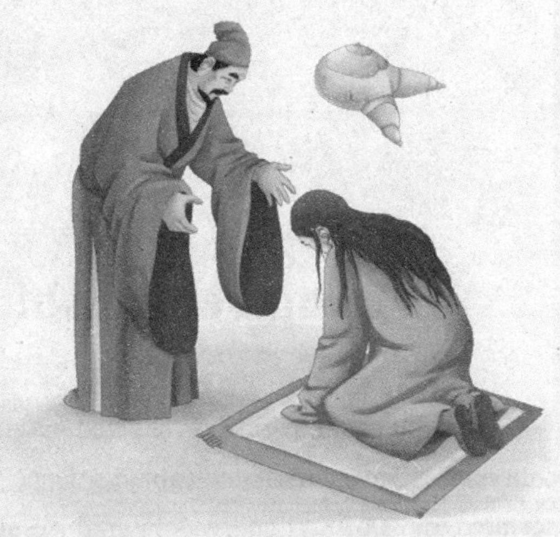

（選自宋 · 洪邁《夷堅志》）

【注釋】

①憫：哀憐。　②凌遲：古代一種分割肢體的酷刑。　③洋州：即今陝西西南部漢水上游的洋縣。

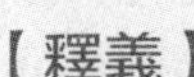

【釋義】

台州監獄中的一個獄吏，十分哀憐一個重囚犯。這個重囚犯很感激他，因而告訴他説：“我七次犯死罪，遭審訊拷打，肺臟大部分受損傷，以至於嘔血。别人傳授給我一個藥方，就是只用白及爲末，每日用米湯沖服，其效如神。”後來這個囚犯被處以極刑，凌遲而死。劊子手將其胸腔剖開，只見肺間數十處受傷造成的孔洞，全部由白及填補起來，其顔色還没有改變。洪貫之聽到這個消息，到洋州上任時，見有一士兵忽然患咯血病，非常危險，他便用此方來救治，一天就止住了咯血。

【按語】

白及，爲多年生草本植物，以其塊莖入藥。這種塊莖，形圓色白，數枚常相連及，故名爲白及。所以《神農本草經》稱爲連及草。

李時珍在《本草綱目·草部》第十二卷“白及”條，引述了洪邁這段記載。時珍説：“白及性澀而收，得秋金之令，故能入肺止血，生肌治瘡也。”並引述宋代蘇頌《本草圖經》

之言："今醫家治金瘡不瘳及癰疽方多用之。"此類病例頗多，不妨再摘録一例。據明代《乘雅》載："杭郡獄中，有犯大辟者，生肺癰，膿成欲死，得單方服白及末，遂獲全生。越十年臨刑，其肺已損三葉，所損處，皆白及末填補，其間形色，猶未變也。"因白及具有收斂止血、消腫生肌的作用，臨床多用於咯血、吐血及外傷出血。近代，常單用本品以糯米湯或凉開水調服，用來治療肺胃出血之症，每獲良效。如獨聖散，即以白及一味調服，治療肺空洞出血，即有特效。

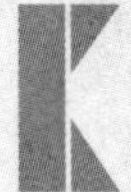

Lung-replenishing Baiji (Bletilla)

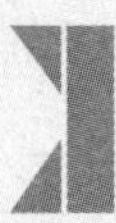

A prison guard in Taizhou showed pity towards a felon. The criminal felt grateful and told him, "I have committed capital offence for seven times. After being interrogated and tortured, most of my lung was injured, resulting in hematemesis. Someone has imparted me an effective repairing method for the lung, which is to take powdered Baiji with rice porridge." Later the criminal was put to death by dismemberment. The executioner cut open his chest, and found holes on his lungs caused by injury were all filled up with Baiji. Hong Guanzhi learnt of it and while he was in Yangzhou, he used the formula to cure a soldier suffering from emptysis.

From *A Collection of Hearsay and Anecdotes*.

Editor's Note:

Baiji is a perennial herb and its roots and stalk can be used as medicine. The roots are round in shape and white in color, often connected in several pieces. Hence the name Baiji or Lianji Cao (meaning "white and connected"). With astringent property, Baiji enters the lung meridian, with effects of arresting blood, generating muscles and healing sores. Clinically it is used to cure hemoptysis, hematemesis and bleeding due to external injury. In modern times, it is often taken together with rice soup or cooled boiled water to treat bleeding of the lung and stomach. It can also be used to cure bleeding of the empty hole in the lung.

【藜蘆愈驚風】

【原文】

一婦病風癇。自七六歲得驚風後，每一二年一作；至五七年，五七作；三十歲至四十歲則日作，或甚至一日十餘作。遂昏癡健忘，求死而已。值歲大饑，采百草食。於野中見草若葱狀，采歸蒸熟飲食。至五更，忽覺心中不安，吐涎如膠，連日不止，約一二斗，汗出如洗，甚昏困。三日後，遂輕健，病去食進，百脈皆和。以所食葱訪人，乃憨葱苗也，即《本草》藜蘆是矣。《圖經》①言能吐風病，此亦偶得吐法耳。

（選自金 · 張子和《儒門事親》卷七）

【注釋】

①《圖經》：指宋代蘇頌主持修訂的《圖經本草》，又称《本草圖經》。

【釋義】

有一婦女患癲癇病。從六七歲時患驚風後，每一兩年發作一次；五七年以後，每年發作五七次；三十歲至四十歲，則每天發作一次，有時甚至每天發作十多次。于是就神志不清，癡呆健忘，痛不欲生。這時正逢大災荒年景，這一病婦只好采野草而食。在野地裏她見到一種類似大葱模樣的野草，就采回蒸熟來填飽肚子。到五更天，忽然覺得心中不舒服，口中流出像膠一樣的涎水，連日不止，約有一二斗，汗出如洗，感到十分困倦。三天後，遂感輕鬆有力，疾病已愈，能進飲食，脈象平和。拿這一婦人所食之物去請教有經驗的人，説這是憨葱幼苗，即《本草》中所説的藜蘆。《本草圖經》中説可以用嘔吐法治風病，這也算是偶然得到的一則土法吧。

【按語】

藜蘆味辛、苦、寒，有劇毒，湧吐風痰、殺蟲。常用於湧吐風痰，治痰涎壅閉之風癇等證。此病例屬痰涎迷塞心竅之症，故遇藜蘆而愈。李時珍在《本草綱目 · 草部》第十七卷“藜蘆”條下，引述了張子和這則病例。

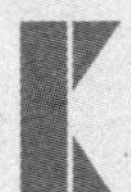

Lilu (Veratrum) Cured Epilepsy

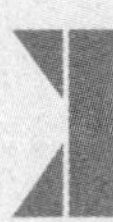

Once there was a woman who suffered from epilepsy when she was six or seven years old. Since then, the disease broke out every other year. Five to seven years later, it broke out five to seven times every year; in her thirties and forties, the disease broke out every day, or even a dozen times every day. Then she lost her mind, with symptoms of amnesia, absent-mindness and aphrenia. She suffered so much that she lost the will to live on. Right then a terrible natural disaster struck the area she lived in. The diseased woman had to collect weeds to eat. Seeing a scallion-like weed in the wilderness, she picked some and steamed it to feed herself. At midnight, she suddenly felt great discomfort, and a significant amount of thick saliva continuously flew out of her mouth. She also sweated a lot and felt exhausted. Three days later, she felt relaxed, energetic, rejuvenated and her appetite was back. Her pulse became mild. What she ate was said to be the sprouts of Hancong, or the so-called Lilu recorded in *King Shen Nong's Classics of Herbal Medicine*. According to *Illustrated Pharmacopoeia*[1], vomiting can be used to treat epilepsy. This was an accidentally obtained vomiting inducement.

From *Instructions on Fulfilling Fillial Piety* (*Rumen Shiqin*).

Notes:

1. *Illustrated Pharmacopoeia* (《本草圖經》Bencao Tujing): It is a groundbreaking work on pharmaceutical botany, zoology, and mineralogy, compiled by Su Song (蘇頌).

Editor's Note:

Lilu is pungent and bitter in flavor, cold-natured, and toxic. With effects of prompting the patient to discharge phlegm and killing parasites, it is used to treat the wind epilepsy due to phlegm-drool stagnation or congestion. This story is a case in point.

甘草解百毒

【原文】

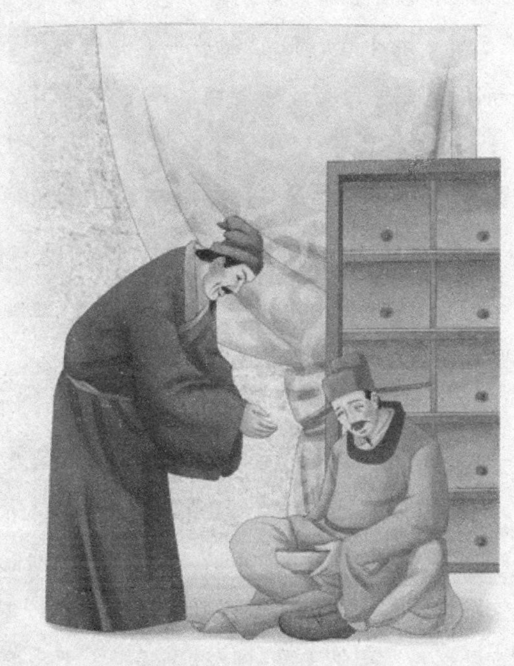

盛御醫寅[①]字啓東，吳江人，少從隱士王賓[②]學醫。永樂[③]中，以解户赴京。後事仁、宣兩朝[④]，皆被眷遇[⑤]。特賜侍以示寵異[⑥]。

他日，寅晨入御藥房，忽頭痛昏眩欲絶，群醫束手，莫知何疾。敕幕人[⑦]療治，有草澤醫人[⑧]請見，投藥一服，逡巡[⑨]却愈。上奇之，召問所用何方。對曰："寅空心入藥室，卒中諸藥之毒，能和諸藥者，甘草也。臣用是爲湯以進耳，非有它術。"上詰寅，果未晨饔[⑩]而入，乃厚勞其人雲。

（選自明 · 陸粲[⑪]《庚巳編》）

【注釋】

①盛御醫寅：即御醫盛寅（1375—1441），字啓東。江蘇吳江縣人，爲名醫戴原禮再傳弟子。曾受明成祖賞識，掌管太醫院事，正統元年 (1436) 返鄉。著有《醫經秘旨》《六經證辨》《流光集》等傳世。 ②隱士王賓：即王仲光，爲儒不仕，學醫道于戴原禮，熟讀《素問》三年，又深研朱彦修醫案，後來名震吳下。③永樂：明成祖朱棣的年號，1403—1424 年。④仁、宣兩朝：即明仁宗、明宣宗兩代皇帝。仁宗朱高熾，年號洪熙，公元 1425 年在位。宣宗朱瞻基，年號宣德，1426—1435 年在位。⑤眷遇：至親相待。⑥賜侍以示寵異：賞賜他的侍從人員而表示寵愛與衆不同。⑦敕 (chì 斥）幕人：命令太醫院的幕賓人等。敕：皇帝的命令。⑧草澤醫人：民間醫生。⑨逡（qūn 群）巡：片刻，須臾。 ⑩饔 (yóng 擁)：指早餐。⑪陸粲：字子餘，一字浚明，吳郡長

洲（今蘇州市）人。生於明孝宗弘治七年（1494年），卒於世宗嘉靖三十年（1551年），享年五十七歲。陸粲少有文名，嘉靖五年中進士。後因捲入統治集團的內部爭鬥，被廷杖下獄，四十歲時，以念母乞歸，裹居凡十八年。陸粲研心經史，學問宏博，著有《陸子餘集》八卷，又有《左傳附註》《春秋胡氏傳辨疑》等，並傳於世。《庚巳編》共十卷，係陸粲早年（即陸粲十六～二十五歲中進士前）所撰筆記。大都爲奇聞異事、因果報應之類，雖多荒誕不經，但從中可發掘出一些可供參考的歷史資料。

【釋義】

御醫盛寅，字啓東，江蘇省吳江市人。少年時拜王賓爲師學醫，永樂年間，奉命攜家調居京城。後來侍奉仁宗、宣宗兩代皇帝，都以至親相待，皇帝特別賞賜他的侍從人員，以表示對他的寵愛與衆不同。

有一天早晨，盛寅剛進御藥房，突然頭痛昏倒，不省人事。太醫院的醫生們，都束手無策，不知何病。皇帝命令幕賓人等急速救治，其中有一民間醫生自薦。他配藥一劑煎湯服下，片刻之間，盛寅竟然蘇醒。皇帝對此感到驚奇，召問服的何藥。草澤醫回答說："盛大人没吃早飯空腹走進藥房，由於胃氣虛懦，中了諸藥之毒，故而昏倒。能解諸藥之毒者，唯有甘草，我是選用甘草一藥濃煎頓服，不是什麼奇方妙藥。"皇帝立即詢問盛寅，果然去藥房時没吃早飯。于是置辦豐厚的禮品，慰勞了這位民間醫生。

【按語】

甘草能調和諸藥，解百毒，故有"國老"之稱。這位草澤醫人，僅用甘草一藥，竟能使御醫盛寅起死回生，即是典型例證。

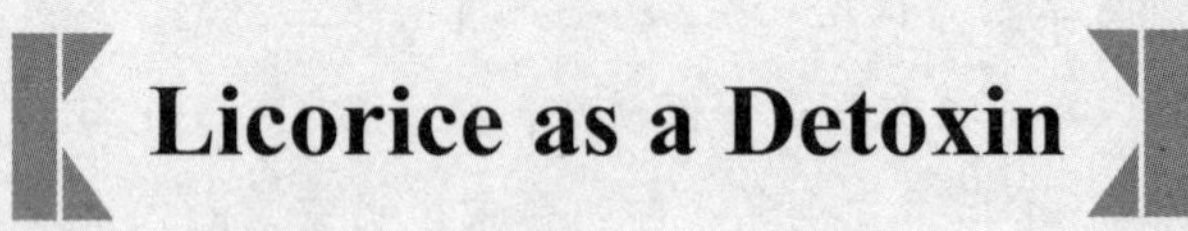

Licorice as a Detoxin

The imperial doctor Sheng Yin was from Wujiang county of Jiangsu Province. He learned medicine from Wang Bin in his childhood. During the reign of Yongle emperor, he was summoned by the court to serve the royalty. He served for Renzong and Xuanzong emperors whole-heartedly. The emperor even awarded his attendants to show a distinctive favor to him.

One day in the morning, when Sheng Yin entered the imperial pharmacy, he suddenly felt a headache and fainted. No one serving in the imperial hospital knew how to treat him. The emperor asked around for a treatment, and then a doctor of low status who had been treating common folks recommended himself to treat Doctor Sheng. He asked the patient to take a particular decoction. Sheng Yin immediately came back to his normal state after taking the medicine. The emperor was impressed and asked the doctor about the prescription. The folk doctor answered, "Mr. Sheng entered the pharmacy probably with an empty stomach, thus fainted after being intoxicated by the smell of all kinds of herbs here. Gancao, or licorice, is an effective detoxin for most drugs, so I just prescribed licorice for him instead of using any complicated formula." The emperor immediately asked Sheng Yin, confirming that he indeed did not have breakfast when he entered the pharmacy. Thus, he granted abundant gifts to the folk doctor.

From *A Collection of Curious Stories*.

Editor's Note:

Gancao can regulate all drugs and relieve numerous toxins, thus was called "Guolao," or the senior among all herbs. The story reveals the medical effects of Gancao.

【菊之本末 罔不有功】

【原文】

菊春生夏茂，秋花冬實，備受四氣①，飽經露霜，葉枯不落，花槁不零②，味兼甘苦，性稟平和。昔人謂其能除風熱，益肝補陰，蓋不知其得金水③之精英尤多，能益金水二臟也。補水所以制火，益金所以平木；木平則風息，火降則熱除。用治諸風頭目④，其旨深微。黄者入金水陰分，白者入金水陽分，紅者行婦人血分，皆可入藥。神而明之，存乎其人。其苗可蔬，葉可啜，花可餌，根實可藥，囊之可枕⑤，釀之可飲，自本至末，罔⑥不有功。宜乎前賢比之君子⑦，神農列之上品⑧，隱士采入酒斝⑨，騷人餐其落英⑩。費長房言九日飲菊酒，可以，辟不祥⑪。《神仙傳》⑫言康風子、朱孺子皆以服菊花成仙。

《荆州記》言胡廣久病風羸，飲菊潭水多壽⑬。菊之貴重如此，是豈群芳可伍⑭哉？

（選自明 ·《本草綱目》卷十五《菊》“發明”）

【注釋】

①四氣：指春、夏、秋、冬四季之氣。②零：凋落。③金水：指秋、冬二季。下句“金水”指肺、腎二臟。④諸風頭目：指因各種風邪所致頭目疾患。⑤囊：裝入口袋。枕：作枕頭。均用作動詞。⑥罔：没有哪一部分。⑦“前賢”六字：三國魏 · 鍾會所撰《菊花賦》有“早植晚發，君子德也”句，故云。⑧“神農”句：《神農本草經》分藥爲三品，菊屬上品，故云。⑨“隱士”句：晋代陶淵明詩文常並言菊與酒，故云。斝（jiǎ甲），古代銅制酒器，似爵而較大。⑩“騷人”句：屈原《離騷》有“夕餐秋菊之落英”句，故云。騷人，詩人，指屈原。⑪“費長房”二句：據南朝梁 · 吴均《續齊諧記》，江南桓景隨費長房游學，長房告之：“九月九日汝家中當有災，急去，令家人各作絳囊，盛茱萸以系臂，登高飲菊花酒，此禍可除。”費長房，東漢方士，《後漢書 · 方術列傳》載其事。九日，指農曆九月初九，亦稱重九、重陽。⑫《神仙傳》：書名。晋代葛洪撰。康風子、朱孺子未見於該書。唐 · 李汾《續神仙傳》卷上言朱孺子爲三國時人，服餌黄精十餘年，後煮食根形如犬、堅硬如石之枸杞，遂升雲而去。⑬《荆州記》二句：據《荆州記》載，胡廣之父患風羸，飲菊潭水而愈。荆州記，晋代盛弘之撰。胡廣，東漢太尉，封育陽安樂鄉侯。⑭伍：同列。

【釋義】

菊春天發芽、夏天繁茂，秋天開花、冬天結籽，完全稟受了四時之氣，飽經了風霜雨露，枝葉枯萎而不落，花朵枯槁而不凋零，味道兼有甘苦，稟性平和不烈。前人説它能除風熱，補益肝陰，大概不知道它稟受秋天冬天的精華更多，能補益肺臟和腎臟。補益腎水是用來制約心火的辦法，補益肺金是用來平息肝木的辦法；肝木平抑肝風就止息，心火下降内熱就消除。用它治療各種風邪引起的頭暈目眩，其意義深奥而微妙。黄菊花入肺、腎二臟的陰分，白菊花入肺、腎二臟的陽分，紅菊花行婦女血分，都可以入藥。只有用心研究的人才能神妙地明察其中的奥理。它的苗可以作爲蔬菜，葉子可以食用，花兒可以吃，根和果實可以入藥，把菊花裝入袋子可以作枕頭，用菊花釀酒可以飲用，從根到梢，没有哪一部分没有功效。難怪前賢把它比作君子，神農把它列入上品，隱士把它采入酒杯，詩人品味它的落花。費長房説九月九喝菊花酒可以消災除禍。《神仙傳》記載康風子、朱孺子都是因爲服食菊花而成仙。《荆州記》説胡廣久患風羸之疾，因爲飲用菊潭水而長壽。菊花如此貴重，這難道是衆花可以相比的嗎？

【按語】

李時珍(1518—1593),字東璧,號瀕湖,蘄州(今湖北省蘄春縣)人。出身中醫世家,明代偉大的醫藥學家。他14歲考中秀才,後三次參加鄉試未中,遂一心習醫,而醫名大震。曾任太醫院院判，後爲修本草而毅然辭職。一生著述甚豐，但大多佚失，唯《本草綱目》大行於世。

《本草綱目》共五十二卷，約一百九十萬字，載藥一八九二種，其中新增藥三七四種，收集醫方一一〇九六首，還繪製了一一六〇幅精美的插圖。該書打破了傳統的上、中、下三品分類法，採用"振綱分目"，科學分類。把藥物分爲礦物藥、植物藥、動物藥。又將礦物藥分爲金、玉、石、鹵四部；將植物藥分爲草、穀、菜、果、木五部；將動物藥按低級向高級進化的順序，分爲蟲、鱗、介、禽、獸、人等六部。每部再細分其目。這種分類法，在當時十分先進。李時珍旁徵博引，並實地考察，根據古籍的記載和自己的親身實踐，對各種藥物的名稱、產地、氣味、形態、栽培、採集、炮製等做了詳細的介紹，並通過嚴密的考證，糾正了前人的一些錯誤。書中涉及內容極爲廣泛，在生物、化學、天文、地理、地質、採礦乃至語言文字和歷史方面都有突出貢獻。這是一部集十六世紀以前中國本草學大成的著作，被譽爲"東方藥物巨典"，英國生物學家達爾文稱《本草綱目》爲"1596年的百科全書"。

1606年,《本草綱目》首先傳入日本；1647年，波蘭人彌格來中國，將其譯成拉丁文流傳歐洲，後來又先後譯成日、朝、法、德、英、俄等文字。

值得一説的是，李時珍嘔心瀝血、殫精竭慮，集二十八年之心血，於1578年他六十一歲時，完成了這部巨著。但由於書中對經典和傳統觀點有冒犯之處，此書一直未能出版。直到十二年後的1590年,南京書商才終於着手刻印。又過了六年,至1596年,該書才正式問世。而李時珍在1593年已長眠地下了。這位偉大的醫學家，生前並沒有看到自己的著作出版，成爲千古憾事。

本文敘述了菊的生長習性及其多方面的作用。指出菊從根到梢，沒有哪一部分沒有功效，一身都是寶，遠非群芳可比。因此，受到歷代文人雅士的推崇。

All Parts of Chrysanthemum are Valuable

Chrysanthemum sprouts in spring, flourishes in summer, blossoms in autumn and produces seeds in winter. Being nurtured by all four seasons, the flower experiences wind, frost, rain and dew, without withering and falling. According to people in the past, it can relieve wind-heat and nourish yin Qi in the liver with bittersweet tastes and mild nature. However, they did not realize that it could tonify the lung and kidney with the essence it absorbs in autumn and winter. Kidney water is nourished to lower excessive heat in the heart; lung metal is nourished to quench liver wood. With quenched liver wood, liver wind will be relieved. With reduced heat in the heart, a person feels cool and refreshed. Using chrysanthemum to treat dizziness caused by different reasons is effective and profoundly challenging.

Yellow chrysanthemum corresponds with the yin division of lung and kidney organs, while white chrysanthemum with the yang division of lung and kidney. Red chrysanthemum is associated with the blood division of women. All of them could be used in prescription. Only people with attentive study could master the secrets and principles. Its seedling could be used as vegetables, and its leaves and flowers edible. Its roots and fruits can be used as drugs. The chrysanthemum blossoms can be filled into bags to form pillows, or dewed in wine to entertain people. Every part from the root to the tip of chrysanthemum has its effect. No wonder the former sages compared it to an ideal Confucian gentleman, King Shen Nong ranked it at the top grade, hermits picked it to take with wine, and poets appreciated it for its fallen flowers. Fei Changfang said that drinking chrysanthemum wine on the ninth of September in the lunar year would keep one away from disasters. According to *Biographies of Divine Immortals* [1], Kang Fengzi and Zhu Ruzi became deities after taking chrysanthemum. According to *Records of Jingzhou*[2], Hu Guang was extremely weak with a chronic disease, but later achieved longevity after drinking chrysanthemum water. How could any other flower be compared to such the valuable chrysanthemum?

From *Compendium of Meteria Medica*[3].

Notes:

1. *Biographies of Divine Immortals* (《神仙傳》 Shenxian Zhuan) : It is a hagiography of “xian” (仙 transcendents or immortals), partially attributed to the Daoist scholar Ge

Hong (283-343).

2. *Records of Jingzhou* (《荆州記》Jingzhou Ji): It is a book written by Sheng Hongzhi (盛弘之) in the Liu Song Dynasty.

3. *Compendium of Materia Medica* (《本草綱目》Bencao Gangmu): It is a Chinese materia medica work written by Li Shizhen in the Ming Dynasty. It is a work epitomizing materia medica in the Ming Dynasty. *Compendium of Materia Medica* is regarded as the most comprehensive medical book ever written in the history of traditional Chinese medicine. It lists all the plants, animals, minerals, and other items that were believed to have medicinal properties. The text consists of 1,892 entries, each entry with its own name called a gang. The mu in the title refers to the synonyms of each name.

Li Shizhen completed the first draft of the text in 1578, after conducting readings of 800 other medical reference books and carrying out nearly 30 years of field study. For this and many other achievements, Li Shizhen is compared to Shennong, a mythological God in Chinese myth who gave instruction on agriculture and herbal medicine.

With the publication of *Compendium of Materia Medica*, not only did it improve the classification of how traditional medicine was compiled and formatted, but it was also an important medium in improving the credibility and scientific values of biology classification of both plants and animals.

The compendium corrected many mistakes and misapprehensions of the nature of herbs and diseases. Li also included many new herbs, adding his own discoveries of particular drugs and their efficacy and function, as well as more detailed descriptions of the results of experiments. It also has notes and records on general medical data and medical history.

Compendium of Materia Medica is also more than a mere pharmaceutical text, for it includes a vast amount of information on topics as wide ranging as biology, chemistry, geography, mineralogy, geology, history, and even mining and astronomy, which might appear to have little connection with herbal medicine. It has been translated into more than 20 languages and spread all over the world. Even now, it is still in print and used as a reference book.

Editor's Note:

The excerpt recorded the life cycle, nature and medical values of chrysanthemums. It pointed out that chrysanthemum was valuable in every part, which was unique among flowers. That is why so many scholars and doctors sang high praise for this type of plant.

【御賜金杵】

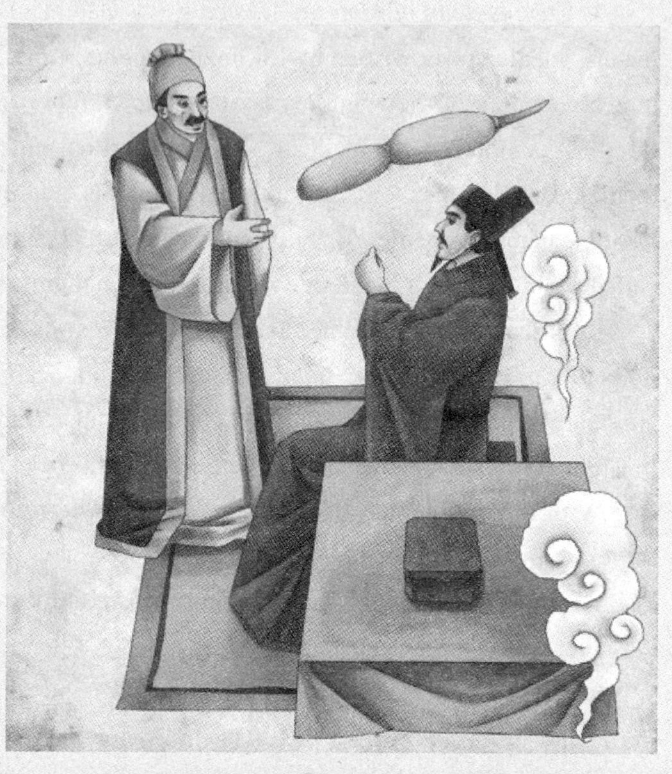

【原文】

宋孝宗[1]患痢，衆醫不效。高宗偶見一小藥肆[2]，召而問之，其人問得病之由，乃食湖蟹所致。遂診脈曰："此冷痢也。"乃用新采藕節搗爛，熱酒調下，數服乃愈。高宗大喜，即以搗藥金杵[3]賜之。

（選自明・李時珍《本草綱目・果部・蓮藕》所引宋・趙溍[4]《養屙漫筆》文）

【注釋】

①孝宗：即宋孝宗趙昚（shèn 慎），宋高宗趙構之子。1163–1189 年在位。②高宗：即宋高宗趙構，1127—1162 年在位。藥肆：藥鋪。③搗藥金杵：用黄金製成的搗藥錘子。④趙溍：南宋學者，生平不詳。所著《養屙漫筆》，系筆記雜談。其中載有數則醫藥資料，多爲民間驗方。

【釋義】

宋孝宗患痢疾，很多御醫治療無效。有一天，宋高宗偶然遇到一家小藥鋪，便召喚鋪主詢問治痢方法。藥鋪先生問發病原因，原來是吃湖裏螃蟹不慎而引起。藥鋪先生診完脈説："這是冷痢呀！"于是用新采湖蓮藕節搗爛取汁，温酒調服。孝宗吃了幾次病就好了。高宗很高興，就把搗藥的金錘賞給了藥鋪先生。

【按語】

本文介紹了用藕節解蟹毒治痢的驗方。據《本草綱目》："藕節，性平，無毒；搗汁飲，主吐血不止、消瘀血、解熱毒，止血痢血崩。"李時珍在引述了趙溍此段文字後説："大抵藕能消瘀血，解熱開胃，而又解蟹毒故也。”所以宋孝宗之病得以速愈，而小藥鋪幸獲御賜金杵。

A Golden Pestle Bestowed by the Emperor

Once Emperor Xiaozong of Song suffered from dysentery, and even the imperial doctors could not solve the problem. One day, his father, Emperor Gaozong came across a drugstore and asked about a treatment of Xiaozong's disease. The drugstore owners asked about the pathogenic reasons and learned that the disease was caused by eating lake crabs. He took Xiaozong's pulse and said, "This is the cold dysentery!" Then he asked people to pick some fresh lotus roots, smash them to produce juice for the emperor to take with warm wine. After taking several doses, Xiaozong recovered. Greatly delighted, Emperor Gaozong awarded the golden pestle used for smashing lotus to the drugstore owner.

From *Compendium of Meteria Medica*.

Editor's Note:

The excerpt introduced a formula of lotus roots that can be used to dissolve crab toxin and treat dysentery. According to *Compendium of Meteria Medica*, lotus root was mild in nature with no toxin. Drinking its juice could cure continuous hematemesis, dissipate blood stasis, relieve heat toxin, arrest dysentery with blood stool and metrorrhagia. That is why the lotus was used to relieve the crab toxin.

【萊菔子消面毒】

【原文】

齊州有人病狂，云夢中見紅裳女引入宮殿中，小姑令歌。每日遂歌云："五靈樓閣曉玲瓏，天府由來是此中。惆悵悶懷言不盡，一丸蘿蔔火吾宮。"有一道士云："此犯大麥毒也。少女心神，小姑脾神。《醫經》言蘿蔔治面毒。故曰火吾宮。火者，毀也。遂以藥並蔔治之，果愈。

（選自明 · 李時珍《本草綱目 · 草部》第二十六卷）

【釋義】

齊州有一個人患癲狂病，説夢中見一個穿紅衣服的少女把他引入宮殿中，一個小姑娘讓他唱歌。于是他每天都唱着："五靈樓閣曉玲瓏，天府由來是此中。惆悵悶懷言不盡，一丸蘿蔔火我宮。"有一個道士説："這是犯了大麥毒的緣故。少女爲心之神，小姑爲脾之神。《醫經》上説蘿蔔治面毒，所以歌聲中説'火我宮'。'火'就是'毀'的意思。"于是就用藥配蘿蔔來進行醫治，果然痊愈。

【按語】

萊菔，亦稱蘆菔，俗稱蘿蔔。種子稱萊菔子，即蘿蔔子。入藥首見於《唐本草》。服用此品，有消谷食、解面毒和祛痰降氣之功效。萊菔，也作來服。來，本義指小麥，像一棵小麥形。由於服用本品有消"來（麥）"食之力，故名來服。宋 · 蘇頌《本草圖經》云：萊菔"尤能制面毒。昔有婆羅門僧東來，見食麥麪者云：'此大熱，何以食之?'又見食中有蘆菔，云賴有此以解其性，自此相傳，食麪必啖蘆菔。"可見萊菔（即蘆菔）消麪食之功。

張錫純《醫學衷中參西録》云："萊菔子無論生或炒，皆能順氣開鬱，消脹除滿。"此例癲狂之病，似爲痰氣上擾清竅，蒙蔽心神所致。藥證相符，故能痊愈。

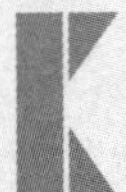

Radish Seeds Cleansing Facial Toxin

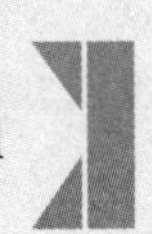

Once in Qizhou there was a person who suffered mental disorder. He told others that he dreamed about being led into a palace by a maiden in red. The maiden asked him to sing everyday, and the lyrics were as follows:

"The five spirits' pavilion is exquisite, with Tianfu originally in between. Words cannot express my melancholy and sadness, a pill of radish fires my palace." A Daoist priest said, "His problem was caused by barley intoxication. The maiden represents his heart energy, while the little girl the spleen energy. According to medical classics, radish can cure facial toxic, thus the song says 'fires our palace', in which fire means destroy." Then he treated the patient with drugs containing radish. After that, the patient recovered.

From *Compendium of Meteria Medica*.

Editor's Note:

Laifu, also called Lufu, is known by common people as radish. Its seeds are called Laifuzi, namely the radish seeds. It can help digest grains, relieve facial toxin, eliminate phlegm and descend qi. Both raw and fried radish seeds can soothe qi, relieve stagnation, distention and fullness. In the clinical case quoted in this story, the conditions were caused by ascending phlegm, thus could be cured with radish seeds.

破故紙壯筋骨

【原文】

破故紙今人多以胡桃合服，此法出自唐鄭相國。自敘云：予爲南海節度，年七十有五，越地卑濕，傷於内外，衆疾俱作，陽氣衰絶，服乳石補藥，百端不應。元和七年[1]，有訶陵國[2]舶主李摩訶，知予病狀，遂傳此方並藥。予初疑而未服。摩訶稽首[3]固請，遂服之。經七八日而覺應驗，自爾常服，其功神效。十年二月，罷郡歸京，録方傳之。

（選自明 · 李時珍《本草綱目 · 草部》第十四卷）

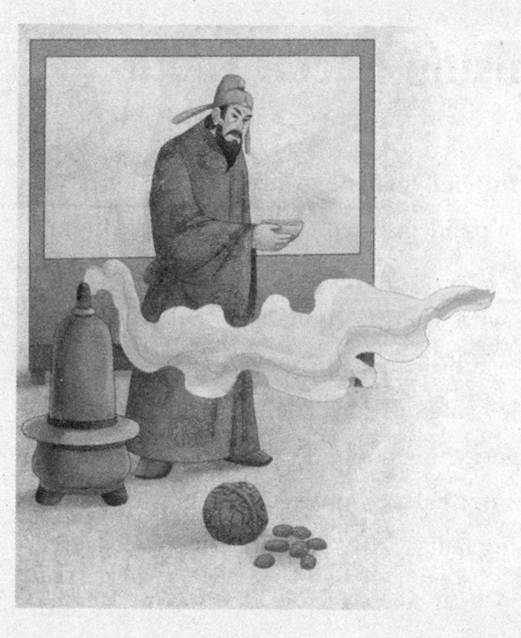

【注釋】

①元和七年：812 年。元和是唐憲宗李純的年號。②訶陵國：即門(shé)婆國。故地在印尼爪哇島和蘇門答臘島。③稽首：古時一種跪拜禮，以頭着地。

【釋義】

現在人們大多把破故紙與胡桃合服，這個藥方出於唐代鄭相國之手。鄭相國自敘説：我任南海節度使時，已七十五歲，南方地勢低而潮濕，體内體外都受侵傷，多種疾病一起發作，陽氣衰絶，服乳石等補藥，都不見效。元和七年，訶陵國的船主李摩訶，瞭解了我的病情，就向我傳授了這個藥方並給予藥物。我開始因有些懷疑而未服用。李摩訶向我施跪拜禮，再三請求，我于是就把藥服下。經七八天後感到有效，自此經常服用，收到神奇的功效。元和十年二月，罷官歸京，記録此方，以傳後世。

【按語】

李時珍在《本草綱目》中，詳細介紹了破故紙方的配製和服用方法："破故紙十兩，净擇去皮，洗過曝，擣篩令細。胡桃瓤二十兩，湯浸去皮，細研如泥。即入前末，更以好蜜和，令如飴糖，瓷器盛之。旦日以暖酒二合，調藥一匙服之，便以飯壓。如不飲酒人，以暖熟水調之。彌久則延年益氣，悦心明目，補添筋骨。但禁芸苔、羊血，餘無所忌。"並説："此方亦可作丸，温酒服之。"又説："此物本自外番隨海舶而來，非中華所有。番人呼爲補骨脂，語訛爲破故紙也。"

補骨脂，爲多年生草本植物的果實，自唐代元和十二年（817 年）始有補骨脂傳入我國的記載。在當時，北方胡人稱作婆固脂，西方番人稱作補骨鴟，俱爲音譯之稱。傳入中原後，婆固脂語訛爲"破故紙"，補骨鴟則訛言爲"補骨脂"。

以上可以看出，中醫藥學在其發展的過程中，是不斷吸收外來民族的有效經驗的。這正體現了華夏民族文化的包容性。

Magical Formula Strengthening Tendons and Bones

Nowadays people often take Poguzhi (Fructus Psoraleae) together with walnuts. This prescription came from Grand counselor Zheng in the Tang Dynasty. Counselor Zheng once said, "When I was appointed the military commissioner guarding the South China sea, I was already seventy-five years old. The southern region has a low altitude and was damp, and my body was damaged internally and externally. Numerous diseases broke out simultaneously, and the yang qi in my body was exhausted. Taking tonics like galaith did not work. In the seventh year of Yuanhe emperor's reign, Captain Li Moke of Heling country learned of my disease and shared with me this prescription and provided me some drugs. At first, I was not sure and did not take it. Li Moke kneeled down to beg me to take it. I thus took the drug and felt its effect after seven to eight days. Since then, I took it often and it worked on me magically. In February of the tenth year of Yuanhe emperor's reign, I resigned and returned to the capital. I am now recording this prescription to pass it on to the later generations."

From *Compendium of Meteria Medica*.

Editor's Note:

The ingredients of Poguzhi and directions of how to take it were recorded in details in *Compendium of Meteria Medica*. Poguzhi, also called Buguzhi, is the fruit of a perennial herb, introduced from overseas. It is used in pills or ground into powder to be taken with wine or warm cooked water. Taking it for a long time can prolong life, invigorate qi, and strengthen tendons and bones. It is incompatible with field mustard and goat's blood. During the development of the traditional Chinese medicine, useful experiences from overseas were often introduced and integrated. This shows the inclusive nature of TCM, and pattern of Chinese culture in general.

【赤小豆治癰瘡】

【原文】

或言共工氏有不才子①，以冬至死爲疫鬼，而畏赤豆，故于是日做赤小豆粥厭②之。亦傅③會之妄説也。又案陳自明《婦人良方》云："予婦食素，産後七日，乳脈不行，服藥無效。偶得赤小豆一升，煮粥食之，當夜遂行，因閲本草載此，謾④記之。"又《朱氏集驗方》云："宋仁宗在東宫時，患痄腮，命道士贊甯治之。取小豆七十粒爲末，傅⑤之而愈。中貴人⑥任承亮後患惡瘡近死，尚書郎傅永授以藥立愈，叩⑦其方，赤小豆也。"予苦⑧脅疽，既至⑨五臟，醫以藥治之甚驗。承亮曰："得非赤小豆耶？"醫謝曰："某用此活三十口，願勿復言。"有僧發背如爛瓜，鄰家乳婢用此治之如神。

此藥治一切癰疽瘡疥及赤腫，不拘善惡，但水調塗之，無不愈者。但其性黏，乾則難揭，入苧根末即不黏，此法尤佳。

（選自明 · 李時珍《本草綱目 · 穀部》第二十四卷）

【注釋】

①不才子：不成器的兒子。②厭：通"壓"。③傅：通"附"。④謾：煩瑣。⑤傅：通"敷"。⑥中貴人：宦官。⑦叩：詢問。⑧苦：以……爲苦。⑨既至：已經侵及。

【釋義】

傳説共工氏有一個不成器的兒子，在冬至這天死去，變爲疫鬼。因爲他畏懼赤小豆，所以，人們在每年的冬至這天煮赤小豆粥來鎮壓他。這只不過是一種牽强附會的荒誕説法。根據陳自明《婦人良方》中記載："我的妻子飲食清素，産後七天，乳汁不下，服藥治療，没有效果。碰巧弄得赤小豆一升，煮成稀粥吃後，當天夜裏乳汁就下來了。翻閲本草書記載赤小豆有這樣功效，因此就煩瑣地做以記録。"又有《朱氏集驗方》中記載："宋仁宗在東宫時，患痄腮，命一個叫贊甯的道士給他治療。用赤小豆七十粒研成細末，調爲糊狀，外敷後，很快就痊愈了。有個叫任承亮的宦官，背部長惡瘡，將要死，尚書傅永給藥治療後，也馬上獲得痊愈。詢問他所用的藥方，原來是赤小豆。"告知説本人因脅部長瘡疽，甚以爲苦，疽毒已侵及内臟，醫生用藥治療後非常效驗。任承亮對那醫生説："你用的藥，莫非是赤小豆吧？"醫生回答説："我用赤小豆爲人治病來養活三十口家人，請求您不要再説。"書中又載：有個僧人患發背瘡像爛瓜一樣，他鄰居家喂乳的婢女用赤小豆給他治療，其效如神，很快就痊愈了。

赤小豆這種藥，能够治療一切癰疽瘡疥和皮膚紅腫，不管病情是在好的階段，還是發展到壞的階段，只需用清水將赤小豆調成糊狀，外塗患處，即可。没有不痊愈的。只是赤小豆性黏，乾後，就難以揭去，加入苧根末就會不黏，這個方法特别好。

【按語】

赤小豆可食可藥。用其煮粥做飯，也是一種香美食品。今之醫者大多用於利濕消腫。綜上所述，可知赤小豆能治療一切癰疽瘡疥及皮膚紅腫，其法便簡，而效神驗。赤小豆又名紅豆，但與同稱紅豆的相思子，迥然不同，因此在使用時應嚴格區别。

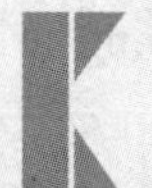

Rice Beans' Medicinal Value

According to an ancient myth, Gonggong had a spoiled son, who died on the coldest day in the winter and became an epidemic demon. He was scared of red beans. Therefore, people kept him under control by cooking red bean porridge on the winter solstice day every year. This was a farfetched and absurd story about red beans. However, red beans do have medicinal values. Chen Ziming wrote in *Compendium of Effective Prescriptions for Women*[1], "My wife often ate vegetables. After giving birth to a baby, she had no breast milk in the first seven days. She took drugs, but they did not work. One day I got some red beans, cooked them into porridge for her to take. The very night she got breast milk. The efficiency of red beans has been recorded in books on materia medica. I would like to confirm it here." *Effective Formulas by Doctor Zhu* also recorded that: When Ren Zong of Song was still a prince and the successor-to-be, he contracted mumps. He ordered a Daoist named Zanning to treat him. Zanning ground seventy pieces of red beans into fine powder and mixed it with water to make some paste. The paste was applied on the prince's face and the prince recovered soon. Later, a eunuch named Ren Chengliang developed malignant carbuncles on the back and was about to die. Fu Yong, an official, prescribed red beans and cured him. Fu Yong once suffered from hypochondriac carbuncles for a long time, the toxin of which had invaded into organs. A doctor treated him effectively. Ren Chengliang asked the doctor, "Was the medicine you used by any chance red beans?"

The doctor answered, "Yes indeed. Red beans are my secret weapons and I have used them to make a living and support my family of thirty. Please let it remain a secret." It was also recorded that a monk whose back carbuncles as big as a rotten watermelon was cured with red beans. The effect was magical and he soon recovered.

Red bean can be used to treat all kinds of carbuncles and swelling. Regardless of the patient's condition, one only needs to make red beans into paste and apply it externally. The patient will certainly recover after that. However, red beans are sticky and hard to remove, so it is nice to add Zhugen (Ramie; Boehmeria) to make it less gluey.

From *Compendium of Meteria Medica*.

Notes:

1. *Compendium of Effective Prescriptions for Women* (《婦人良方》Furen Liangfang): It is a treatise on obstetrics and gynecology, compiled by Chen Ziming in the Song Dynasty.

Editor's Note:

Red bean is edible and also can be used as medicine. Made into porridge or taken as a drug, it will induce diuresis and dissipate swelling. It is also simple and effective to use red beans to treat all kinds of carbuncles, boils and swelling. Red beans should not be confused with Xiangsizi (love pea seed), which is sometimes also called "red beans" . The two should be strictly differentiated.

【劉寄奴草】

【原文】

宋高祖[1]劉裕，小字寄奴。微時伐荻新洲[2]，遇一大蛇，射之。明日往，聞杵臼聲。尋之，見童子數人皆青衣，于榛林中搗藥。問其故，答曰："我主爲劉寄奴所射，今合藥傅[3]之。"裕曰："神何不殺之？"曰："寄奴王者，不可殺也。"裕叱[4]之，童子皆散，乃收藥而反。每遇金瘡傅之即愈，人因稱此草爲寄奴草。鄭樵《通志》[5]云："江南人因漢[6]時謂劉爲卯金刀，乃呼劉爲金。"是以又有金寄奴之名，江東人謂之烏藤菜云。

（選自明 · 李時珍《本草綱目 · 草部》第十五卷）

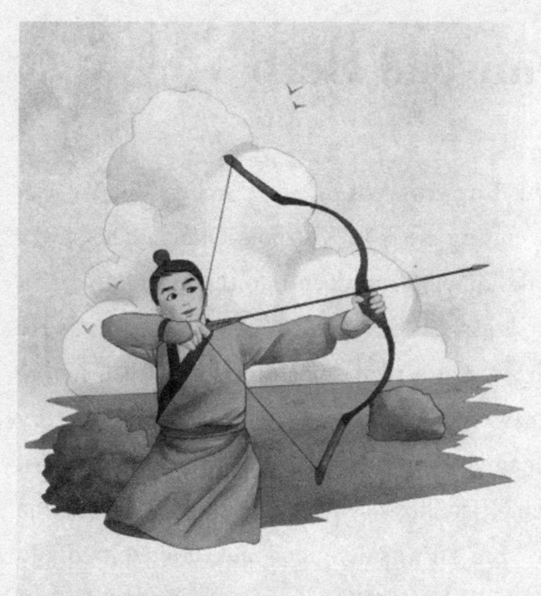

【注釋】

①宋高祖：據史料記載，應爲“宋武帝”。②新洲：南朝梁置。明廢。今廣東省新興縣。③傅：通“敷”。④叱：大聲喝斥。⑤鄭樵：字漁仲，福建莆田人，官至樞密院編修。南宋著名學者。所著《通志》是一部紀傳體的通史，上自三皇，下至唐代，體例略同《史記》。記載各個朝代的重要史實和典章制度。⑥漢：當爲“宋”。

【釋義】

劉寄奴是宋武帝劉裕的小名，劉裕小時候家裏很窮，在新洲靠割茅草爲生。一天，看見一條大蛇，用箭射中，大蛇迅速向茅草深處游去。第二天，又到原處割草時，聽到附近有搗臼之聲，他循聲查找，發現幾個穿青布衣服的童子，在搗一種鮮草藥。劉裕問其故，答道：“昨天，我家主人被一個叫劉寄奴的射了一箭，傷勢不輕，我等在爲主人搗藥。”劉裕又問他們：“神爲何不殺掉劉寄奴呢？”這些童子説：“劉寄奴將來要做皇帝，不可殺”。劉裕心裏很高興，于是，大喝一聲，把這些童子嚇得一哄而散。劉裕便把這些草藥拿回家去，每遇外傷，就用此藥敷之即愈。後人就把此草藥稱爲“劉寄奴草”。南宋鄭樵在《通志》中説“江南人因宋時諱劉爲‘卯金刀’，乃呼‘劉’爲‘金’。”故有金寄奴之名，而江東人又常謂之烏藤菜。

【按語】

劉寄奴，爲菊科草本植物的全草。此草最初由南朝宋武帝劉寄奴所發現，並以其治療金瘡，故後人將此草稱爲劉寄奴草。李時珍的這段記載，來自《南史》第一卷《宋武帝本紀》，又做了一些文字加工，使故事更加完整。文末又引用南宋鄭樵《通志》之語，説明劉寄奴又稱“金寄奴”的緣由。

因劉寄奴草有破血通經、散瘀止痛之功效，故常用於血滯經閉、産後瘀血腹痛、折跌損傷及創傷出血等證。又因爲劉寄怒草氣味芳香，有醒脾開胃、消食化積之功效，故又稱“化食丹”。

Diverse Wormwood Herb

Liu Jinu was the infant name of Liu Yu, Emperor Wu of Song. When Liu Yu was young, his family was poor, and he lived by cutting grass in Xinzhou. One day, he saw a big snake and shot it with an arrow. The snake quickly ran deep into the grass. The next day, when he went to the same place to cut grass, he heard the sound of pounding. He traced the sound and found several boys dressed in green smashing some fresh herbs. Liu Yu asked about the reason. The boys answered, "Yesterday our master was shot by a man named Liu Jinu. He was severely damaged. We're making drugs for him." Liu Yu then asked them, "Why didn't he kill Liu Jinu?" The boys said, "Liu Jinu will become the emperor one day, thus he shouldn't be killed." Liu Yu was delighted and shouted loudly to scare the boys away. Liu Yu then brought the drugs home. Whenever he suffered an injury or wound, he would apply the drug and then recover. People later called the drug "Liu Jinu Herb (Diverse Wormwood Herb, *Herba Artrmisiae Anomalae*)" . Zheng Qiao in the Southern Song Dynasty recorded in *A Comprehensive Collection of Notes and Records*[1], "People living on the southern side of the Yangtze River called it Jin Jinu because of the association of Liu with the Jin radical." In addition, people living on the southern side of the Yangtze River called it "Wuteng Cai" .

From *Compendium of Meteria Medica*.

Notes:

1. *A Comprehensive Collection of Notes and Records* (《通志》Tong Zhi) : It is a biographic comprehensive history book written by Zheng Qiao in the Southern Song Dynasty.

Editor's Note:

Liu Jinu, an herb of the composite family, was said to be found by Emperor Liu Jinu in the Southern Song Dynasty. It was first used to cure incised wound. Because of its effects of regulating blood and menstruation, scattering stasis and arresting pain, it was often used to treat blood stagnation, amenorrhea, postnatal blood stasis, abdominal pain, traumatic injury and bleeding. Besides, the fragrant herb also has the effects of activating the functions of spleen and stomach, promoting digestion and relieving food retention. Therefore, it is also called Huashi Dan (Digestive Pills).

【何首烏】

【原文】

此藥本名交藤，因何首烏服而得名也。唐元和[①]七年，僧文象遇茅山[②]老人，遂傳此事。李翱乃著《何首烏傳》云："何首烏者，順州南河縣人。祖名能嗣，父名延秀。能嗣本名田兒，生而閹弱，年五十八無妻子，常慕道術隨師在山。一日醉卧山野，忽見有藤二株，相去三尺餘，苗蔓相交，久而方解，解了又交。田兒驚訝其異，至旦遂掘其根歸，問諸人，無識者。後有山老忽來，示之，答曰："子既無嗣，其藤乃異，此恐是神仙之藥，何不服之？"遂杵爲末，空心酒服一錢，七日而思人道，數月似强健，因此常服。又加至二錢，經年舊疾皆痊，髮烏容少。十年之内，即生數男，乃改名能嗣。又與其子延秀服，皆壽百六十歲。延秀生首烏，首烏服藥，亦生數子，年百三十歲，髮猶黑。有李安期者，與首烏鄉里親善，竊得方服，其壽亦長，遂敘其事傳之云。

（選自明 · 李時珍《本草綱目 · 草部》第十八卷）

【注釋】

①元和：憲宗（李純）的年號。②茅山：原稱句曲山。在江西省西南部，地跨句容、金壇等縣境。

【釋義】

此藥原名叫交藤，因爲何首烏經常服用這個藥，于是就將它稱作何首烏。唐代元和七年，有個叫文象的僧人，遇見了茅山老人，遂把何首烏的故事傳了下來。李翱就寫了《何首烏傳》：何首烏是順州南河縣人，祖父叫能嗣，父名叫延秀。能嗣本來的名字叫田兒，生來就虚弱多病，年已五十八歲，尚無妻室兒女，經常羨慕道家方術，隨同老師入山中修道。一天喝醉了酒睡在山野之中，忽然看見有藤蔓二株，相距三尺多遠，苗蔓相纏，良久才分開，如此反復纏繞相交。田兒看了異常驚奇，到天明即挖去此藤的根回家，問之於人，皆不認識。後來有一位山中老人忽然來到，看後説"你既然無嗣育，這藤如此異常，恐怕是神仙之藥，爲何不把它服下去？"于是就把藥搗碎爲末，空腹用酒冲服一錢，七天就有性欲的要求，過了數月後，自覺身體健壯。因此就常常服這藥。後又將藥量加至二錢。過了一年後，原來身上的疾病也痊愈了，頭髮也多變黑了，面容也年輕了許多。十年之内，就生了幾個男孩，于是就改名叫“能嗣”。又把這個藥給其子延秀吃，結果他們的壽限都活到一百六十歲。延秀生首烏，首烏服此藥，也生了幾個兒子，活到一百三十歲，頭髮仍然烏黑。有個叫李安期的人，與首烏同爲鄰居，相處也很親近，他竊得此方，其壽命也延長了許多，遂將此事記載而傳下來。

【按語】

李翺（772—841）：唐代趙郡人，曾從韓愈學文，爲唐代著名的文學家和哲學家。考李翺《何首烏傳》，與李時珍所引述的這篇《何首烏傳》，雖然内容基本相同，但文字多有出入。至宋代嘉祐年間，蘇頌在李翺所傳的基礎上，又爲何首烏寫了一篇新傳，收在《本草圖經・何首烏》中。内容稍加删減。因篇幅所限，在此不便羅列。將李翺、蘇頌和李時珍三家之文相比較，可知李時珍是將唐、宋時期流傳的《何首烏傳》融爲一體，經過加工整理，使其情節更加完善。

何首烏録作藥用，最早見於五代時成書的《日華子本草》。在宋初的《開寶本草》中，述論了何首烏的功效：“益氣血、黑髭髮，悦顔色，久服長筋骨，益精髓，延年不老。”之後，歷代本草及其他著作所述漸多。近代藥理研究證實，何首烏具有降低血脂、膽固醇和血糖的作用，並有顯著的强心功能。單服何首烏，對腦動脈硬化、冠心病有預防作用。

Fleeceflower Root

The drug was originally called Jiaoteng and later called Heshouwu (Fleeceflower Root, *Radix Polygoni Multiflori*) since a person named He Shouwu was among the first to take the drug. In the seventh year of Yuanhe emperor's reign in the Tang Dynasty, a monk named Wenxiang met an old man in Maoshan, learned of Heshouwu's story and passed it down. Later, Li Ao wrote the story in *Biography of Heshouwu* (《何首烏傳》Heshouwu Zhuan). Heshouwu lived in Nanhe prefecture of Shunzhou. His grandfather was named Nengsi (literally "able to produce offspring)" , and his father Yanxiu (literary "to continue the refined essence"). Nengsi was originally named Tian'er, and had been weak since his birth. When he was fifty-eight years old, he still had no wife or children. He often admired the Daoist approach to immortality and went deep into the mountain to learn the Daoist way and to cultivate his mind. One day he was drunk and slept in wilderness. Suddenly he saw two intertwining vines. Surprised and curious, Tian'er dug out the vine's root in the next morning and took it home. He enquired other people about the vine but nobody knew about it. Later an old man went there unexpectedly and said, "Since you have no children and encountered this plant by accident, maybe it is a remedy from heaven. Why not take the extraordinary herb?" Hearing this, Tian'er smashed the herb into powder, took it with wine on empty stomach. Seven days later, he had sexual desire; and months later, he felt strong and robust. Since then he often took the drug and later increased the dosage. After a year, he fully recovered from physical weakness, his hair growing with a shine, and his face with a healthy glow. He had several sons within ten years, and thus changed his name into Nengsi. Later, he asked his son Yanxiu to take the drug. They all lived until 160 years old. Yanxiu has a son named Shouwu, who also had several sons and lived until 130 years old, when his hair was still black. A man named Li Anqi was one of Shouwu's neighbours and was close to him. He stole the secret prescription and extended his longevity. Later, he recorded the story.

From *Compendium of Meteria Medica*.

Editor's Note:

He Shouwu is medicated to nourish Qi and blood, strengthen tendons and bones, enrich the essence and prolong life. People who take it can keep their hair black and complexion refined. According to recent pharmaceutical research, Heshouwu can reduce fat in the blood, cholesterol level and blood sugar, and tonify the heart. It is also taken to prevent cerebral arteriosclerosis and coronary heart disease.

【威靈仙治痹】

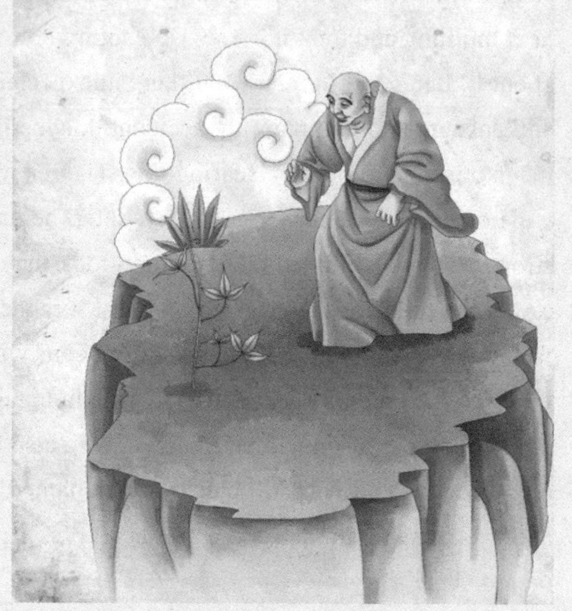

【原文】

先時，商州有人病手足不遂，不履地者數十年。良醫殫[1]技莫能療，所親置之道旁，以求救者。遇一新羅[2]僧見之，告曰："此疾一藥可活，但不知此土有否？"因爲之入山求索，果得，乃威靈仙也。使服之，數日能步履。其後山人[3]鄧思齊知之，遂傳[4]其事。

（選自明·李時珍《本草綱目·草部》第十八卷）

【注釋】

①殫（dān 單）：竭盡。 ②新羅：朝鮮古國名。 ③山人：舊指隱士。 ④傳（zhuàn 賺）：記載。

【釋義】

古時候，商州有一個人患半身不遂，不能走路已數十年。許多有名的醫生用盡了醫術也治不好，他的親人把他放在路旁，以求能救治的人。一個新羅國的和尚路過這裏看見了，告訴他說："這種病有一種藥可以治好，但不知這地方有没有。"于是和尚爲救這位病人就上山找藥，果然找到了，就是威靈仙。便讓他服用，僅數日便能走路，後來隱士鄧思齊知道了，就把這件事記載了下來。

【按語】

威靈仙性急善走，味辛，散風，除濕。此病例顯然系風濕引起的癱瘓，故能生效。

Chinese Clematis Root Cured Physical Impediment

In the past, there was a person in Shangzhou, who suffered from paralysis. He had not been able to walk for decades. Many famous doctors had exhausted their resources and knowledge but still could not cure him. His relatives put him on the roadside with the slim hope that someone would come with a magical cure. When a monk from Xinluo (current day Korea) passed by, he told the patient, "This disease can only be cured with one drug, which may not be found here." The monk then went into the mountain to look for the herb, Weilingxian (Chinense Clematis Root, *Radix Clematidis*), and finally found it. After taking the drug for several days, the patient could walk. Later, a hermit named Deng Siqi learned of this story and kept it in records.

From *Compendium of Meteria Medica.*

Editor's Note:

Weilingxian is pungent in flavor, with an effect of dissipating wind cold and relieving dampness. The patient's problem in the story is probably paralysis caused by rheumatism, thus could be cured by this particular herb.

蒸餅止淋

【原文】

宋寧宗[①]爲郡王時，病淋，日夜凡三百起。國醫罔措，或舉孫琳治之。琳用蒸餅、大蒜、淡豆豉三物搗丸，令以温水下三十丸。曰：今日進三服。病當減三分之一，明日亦然，三日病除。已而果然。賜以千緡[②]。

（選自明 · 李時珍《本草綱目 · 穀部》第二十五卷引《愛竹談藪》）

【注釋】

①宋寧宗：趙擴，1194—1224 年在位。②緡：穿錢的繩子，亦指成串的錢，一千文爲一緡。

【釋義】

宋寧宗作郡王的時候，患淋病，一晝夜要起來小便多次。朝中名醫都束手無措。有人舉薦孫琳去給他醫治。孫琳用蒸餅、大蒜、淡豆豉三味藥物搗爛爲丸。讓他用温水服下三十丸，並告訴他説："今日服三次，病當減三分之一，明日也是這樣，三天病就會痊愈。"後來病果然好了，郡王賞賜孫琳千緡錢幣。

【按語】

蒸餅，味甘，平，無毒。主治消食，養脾胃，温中化滯，益氣和血，止汗，利三焦，通水道。時珍曰："小麥麵修治食品甚多，惟蒸餅其來最古，是酵糟發成單面所造，丸藥所須，且能治痰，而本草不載，亦一缺也。"

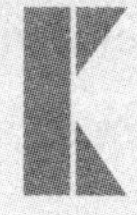

Steamed Pancake Cured Gonorrhea

When Emperor Ning of Song was still a prince, he suffered from gonorrhea and had to urinate multiple times in a day. Many famous doctors had no idea how to treat his disease. Someone recommended Sun Lin. Sun smashed steamed pancake, garlic and fermented soybean into pills and asked the prince to take thirty pills with warm water, telling him that with this formula his conditions would be relieved very day, and he would recover in three days. Later the patient indeed fully recovered. The prince thus awarded thousands of strings of coins to Sun Lin.

From *Compendium of Meteria Medica*.

Editor's Note:

Steamed pancake is sweet in flavor, mild in property and non-toxic. It is mainly used to smooth the digest system, including spleen and stomach. Its main effects include warming the inner organs, dissolving stagnation, nourishing qi, regulating blood, stop sweating, etc. According to Li Shizhen, steamed pancakes were made of fermented flour and used to eliminate phlegm.

【鶉消鼓脹】

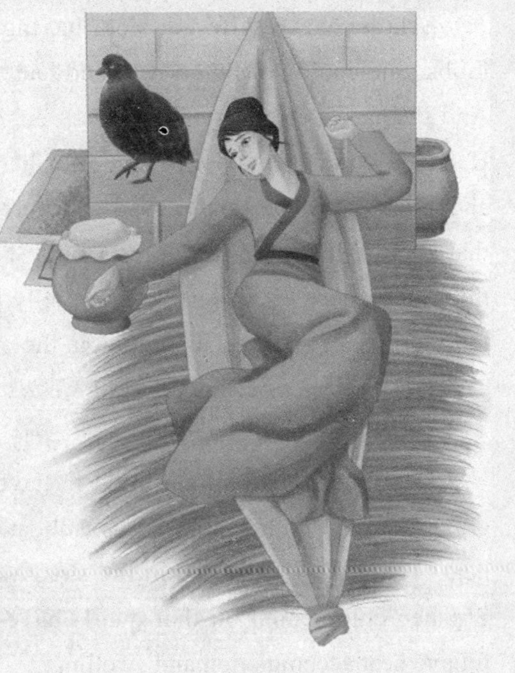

【原文】

魏秀才妻，病腹大如鼓，四肢骨立，不能貼席，惟衣被懸卧，穀食不下者數日矣。忽思鶉食，如法進之，遂運劇。少頃雨汗，莫能言，但有更衣①狀。扶而圊②，小便突出白液，凝如鵝脂。如此數次，下盡遂起。此蓋中焦濕熱積久所致也。

（選自明 · 李時珍《本草綱目 · 禽部》第四十八卷引《董炳集驗方》）

【注釋】

①更衣："大便"的委婉語。　②圊（qīng 青）：厠所。

【釋義】

魏秀才的妻子，患病腹大如鼓，四肢皮包骨頭，不能貼近床席，只好裹了被子懸立着睡覺，已有數日未進飲食。她忽然想吃鶉肉，家人就做好了讓她吃。于是腹内蠕動劇烈，停了一會兒汗流如雨，雖不能説話，但有想解手之狀。就攙扶她去厠所，突然小便下白色液體，凝結如鵝油，像這樣小便了數次，一直把腹内的積液下盡，病就好了。這大概是中焦濕熱積聚時間太長所造成的吧。

【按語】

鶉肉味甘平，無毒。能補五臟，益中續氣，實筋骨，耐寒暑，消積熱。魏秀才之妻所患之病系中焦濕熱積聚所致。在引述此病例後，時珍謹按："鶉乃蛙化，氣性相同，蛙與蛤蟆皆解熱治疳，利水消腫；則鶉之消鼓脹，蓋亦同功云。"

Consuming Quail Meat to Relieve Distention

Scholar Wei's wife got sick, having a belly bulging like a big drum and skinny limbs. She could not lie on bed, and had to be wrapped by a quilt and hanged to sleep. And she hadn't eaten anything for several days. One day she suddenly craved quail meat. Her family members cooked some for her to eat. After eating the meat, she felt intense abdominal peristalsis and perspired severely. Though she could not speak, she indicated that she wanted to go to the restroom. She urinated white liquid, which was dense and thick like goose oil. After that, her belly became flat. What she had before was due to long-term damp-heat accumulation in the middle part of her body.

From *Compendium of Meteria Medica*.

Editor's Note:

Quail meat is sweet and mild in flavor and non-toxic. It can nourish the five inner organs, enrich the essential qi, consolidate tendons and bones and relieve the excessive heat. The patient's disease in the story was due to the accumulation of damp heat. Li Shizhen commented on that quails have similar property with frogs, and both could relieve heat accumulation and swelling.

螢火武威丸

【原文】

昔漢冠軍將軍武威太守劉子南，從道士尹公受得此方。永平十二年①，於北界與虜戰敗績，士卒略盡②，子南被圍，矢下如雨，未至子南馬數尺，矢輒墜地。虜以爲神，乃解去。子南以方教子弟，爲將皆未嘗被傷也。漢末青牛道士得之，以傳安定皇甫隆，隆以傳魏武帝，乃稍③有人得之。故一名冠軍丸，又名武威丸。

（選自明 · 李時珍《本草綱目 · 蟲部四十一卷》引《神仙感應篇》）

【注釋】

①永平十二年：69 年。永平是東漢明帝劉莊的年號。②略盡：大致殆盡。③稍：

漸漸。

【釋義】

從前，漢朝的冠軍將軍，武威府的太守劉子南，從道士尹公那裏得到了配製螢火丸的藥方。永平十二年，劉子南在北部邊疆與外族打仗失敗，士兵差不多犧牲完了。劉子南被敵人圍困，射來的箭像雨點一樣的密，但還没到劉子南的馬數尺的地方，箭就墮落地下。敵人認爲這是神仙之力，於是就撤兵解圍。劉子南把這個藥方教給他的弟子，帶兵打仗都不曾受過傷。漢朝末年青牛道士得到這個藥方，就把它傳授給皇甫隆，皇甫隆又傳給了魏武帝（曹操），以後就逐漸有人得到這個藥方了。所以，螢火丸一名冠軍丸，又名武威丸。

【按語】

螢火即飛螢。味辛，微温，無毒。能明目，療青盲。主治小兒火瘡傷，熱氣蠱毒等。至於所引《神仙感應篇》記載螢火丸之文，蒙上一層神秘色彩，未免太誇張。但關於螢火丸之功效，古代醫家多有描述。北宋龐安常《傷寒總病論》云："曾試用之，一家五十餘口俱染疫病，惟四人帶此者不病也。"極言其效驗。南宋傷寒大家許叔微在《傷寒歌》中亦稱贊之。李時珍在《本草綱目》中説："予亦恒欲試之，因循未暇耳。"爲何會有如此功效呢？還是李時珍一語道破實質："螢火能辟邪明目，蓋取其照幽夜明之義耳。"

Powerful Firefly Pill

In ancient times, the champion general in the Han Dynasty, Liu Zinan in Wuwei Prefecture, got a prescription of Yinghuo Wan (Firefly pill). In the twelfth year of Yongping emperor's reign, Liu Zinan was losing a battle to the nomadic tribes coming from outside the northern border. Almost all soldiers died, and the enemy surrounded Liu Zinan. Arrows were targeted at him, dense like raindrops, but all fell onto the ground before reaching a certain distance away from his horse. Thinking it was the divine intervention, the enemy quickly withdrew. Liu Zinan then passed the prescription to his disciples, which protected them from being hurt in battles. A Daoist at the end of the Han

Dynasty got the prescription and passed it on to Huangfu Long, and Huangfu to Emperor Wu Di of Wei (Cao Cao[1]). Later, other people got the prescription. Therefore, Yinghuo Wan (Firefly pill) was also called Guanjun Wan (Champion pill), or Wuwei Wan (pill from the Wuwei Prefecture).

From *Compendium of Meteria Medica.*

Notes:

1. Cao Cao: (155 – 220), one of the main political figures during the Three Kingdoms Period (220 – 280 AD).

Editor's Note:

Firefly is pungent in flavor, slightly warm in property and non-toxic. It can be used to brighten eyes, treat eyesight loss, pediatric burns and intoxication. Though the excerpt was a little exaggerated and legendary, firefly pills were indeed widely used in Chinese history.

【石龍芻】

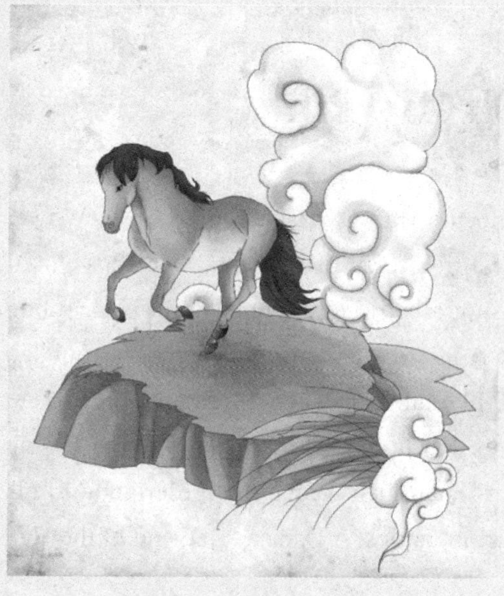

【原文】

周穆王東海島中養八駿處，有草名龍芻，是矣。故古語云："一束龍芻，化爲龍駒。"亦孟子芻豢①之義，龍鬚、王母簪，因形也。縉雲②，縣名，屬今處州，仙都山産此草，因以名之。崔豹《古今注》云："世言黃帝乘龍上天，群臣攀龍鬚墜地生草，名曰龍鬚者，謬也。江東以草織席，名西王母席，亦豈西王母騎虎而墮其須乎？"

（選自明 · 李時珍《本草綱目 · 草部》第十五卷引《述異記》）

【注釋】

①芻豢:《孟子・告子上》:"故理義之悦我心，猶芻豢之悦象口。"朱熹注:"草食曰芻，牛羊是也；穀食曰豢，犬豕是也。"此泛指家畜。②縉云:縣名，今屬浙江省。

【釋義】

周穆王在東海島中養八匹駿馬的地方，有一種草叫龍芻，就是這種草。所以古語說:"一束龍芻，化爲龍駒。"這就是孟子所說的家畜的意思。龍鬚、王母簪，是因其形狀相似而取名的。縉雲，是一個縣名，屬於處州的轄區，這裏的仙都山産這種草，因此把它又命名爲縉雲草。崔豹在《古今注》中說:"世人流傳説，黄帝乘龍上天，群臣都拉着龍鬚，龍鬚墜地生成草，所以，稱這種草爲龍鬚草，這是一種荒謬的説法。如江東用草編席，名叫西王母席，這難道就是西王母騎虎而墮落的虎須嗎?"

【按語】

石龍芻又名龍鬚草、草續斷、縉雲草。時珍曰:"刈草包束曰芻。此草生水石之處，可以刈束養馬，故謂之龍芻。"所引《述異記》之文，是關於石龍芻命名的神話故事，自不必細究。但石龍芻治病之功不可掩。《神農本草經》將其列入上品。《本草綱目》説:"主治心腹邪氣，小便不利淋閉，久服補虛羸，輕身，耳目聰明，延年。"

Shilong Chu
(Stone-side Feeding Grass)

There was a type of grass named Longchu in the eastern sea, where King Mu of Zhou raised eight distinguished horses. Hence an ancient saying "Longchu feeds and produces imperial horses" . Longchu had a variety of names, including Longxu (Dragon's moustache) and Wangmu Zan (Empress' hairpin), which were both descriptive of its shape. It was also named Jinyun Cao (grass) because it was produced in Xiandu Mountain of Jinyun County. Cui Bao said in *Notes of Ancient and Current Times*[1], "It is generally acknowledged that the Yellow Emperor went up to the heaven by riding the dragon. Then all the ministers pulled the dragon's moustaches, which fell onto the ground and became grass. Thus the grass was named Longxu Cao (Dragon's moustache grass). This was obviously a legend. The grass-weaved mat in Jiangdong was called Western Empress's mat. It cannot be made of the moustache of tiger ridden by the Western Empress, can it?"

From *Compendium of Meteria Medica*.

Notes:

1. *Notes of Ancient and Current Times* (《古今注》Gujin Zhu): It is a book written by Cui Bao in the Jin Dynasty, explaining various things and incidents people had heard of from the past to present.

Editor's Note:

Found in water or beside rocks, this herb can be used to feed horses, thus was also called Shi Longchu (Stone-side feeding grass). According to *Compendium of Materia Medica*, the herb was used to treat problems within the heart and abdomen, disinhibit urine, boost the energy and prolong one's life.

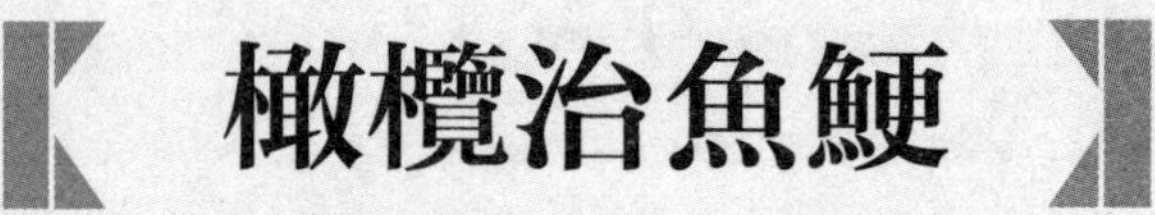

【原文】

吳江一富人，食鱖魚①被鯁，横在胸中，不上不下，痛聲動鄰里，半月餘幾②死。忽遇漁人張九，令取橄欖與食。時無此果，以核研末，急流水調服，骨遂下而愈。

（選自明 · 李時珍《本草綱目 · 果部》第十三卷引《名醫録》）

【注釋】

①鱖（guì 貴）魚：亦稱“桂魚”。是我國名貴淡水食用魚之一。②幾：幾乎。

【釋義】

吳江有一富人，因吃鱖魚，被魚刺卡着嗓子，横在胸口處，不上不下，痛苦的喊叫聲驚動了鄰里，半個多月後，幾乎病死。一個偶然的機會，遇到一個打魚人名叫張九，他讓拿橄欖來吃。當時無橄欖果，就用橄欖核研末，用河中的急流水調服，魚骨立即被冲下而獲痊愈。

【按語】

橄欖產於南方，《本草綱目》曰："氣味酸、甘、温，無毒，主治：生食、煮飲，並消酒毒，解鯸鮐魚毒。嚼汁咽之，治魚鯁。"可見，此例藥症相符，故得痊愈。

Olive Used to Treat Choke on Fishbone

Once there was a rich man in Wujiang. When he ate the mandarin perch, he choked on a piece of fishbone. It could not be taken out or swallowed, which made him quite painful. He cried so loudly that he disturbed the neighbors, and he nearly died. One day, he came across a fisherman named Zhang Jiu. The fisherman asked him to eat olives. Since there was no olive in that season, he ground olive cores into powder and took them with water from a running stream. Then the fishbone was rushed down and the patient recovered.

From *Compendium of Meteria Medica.*

Editor's Note:

Found in the South China, olive is sour and sweet in flavor, warm in nature and non-toxic. Raw or cooked olives are both used as detoxin after one had two much wine or fugu fish. Chewing and swallowing the juice can rescue one from the choke on fish bone.

【胡王使者】

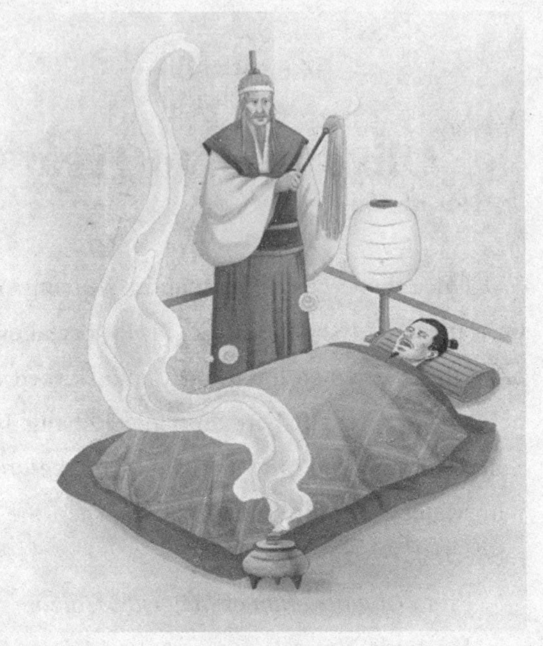

【原文】

唐劉師貞之兄病風[①]。夢神人曰:"但取胡王使者,浸酒服便愈。"師貞訪問,皆不曉。復夢其母曰:"胡王使者[②],即羌活也。"求而用之,兄疾遂愈。

(選自明・李時珍《本草綱目・草部》第十三卷)

【注釋】

①病風:患風濕病。 ②胡王使者:羌活別名。

【釋義】

唐代劉師貞的兄長患風濕病,夜夢神人指點説:"只需取胡王使者泡酒服用便能治愈。"師貞到處問,都不知道什麼是胡王使者。後又夢見他的母親説:"胡王使者,就是羌活。"劉師貞將羌活求來用之,他兄長的風濕病很快就治好了。

【按語】

胡王使者是羌活的別名,因產于古代北國胡地故有此稱。因羌活一莖直上,不爲風摇,故又名獨活。因此草得風不摇,無風自動,故又名獨摇草。性味,辛、苦、温,能發散風寒,通痹止痛。故此例風濕病得以治愈。文中托夢之説,僅是一種形式而已。

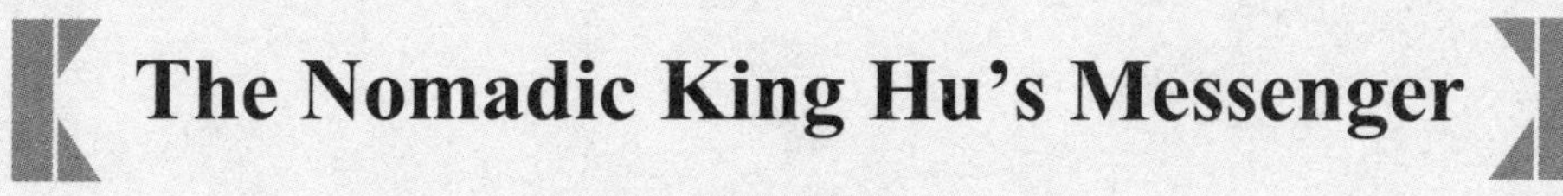

The Nomadic King Hu's Messenger

The elder brother of Liu Shizhen in the Tang Dynasty suffered from rheumatism. He dreamed of being instructed by a deity, who said, "If you want to cure your brother, just ask him to take the medicine called 'Nomadic King's messenger." Liu inquired many people, but no one knew what was the messenger of the Nomadic King. Then he dreamed of his mother, who told him that "Nomadic King's messenger" meant Qianghuo (Notopterygium root, Rhizoma seu Radix Notopterygii). Liu Shizhen found some Qianghuo for his elder brother, who then recovered soon.

From *Compendium of Meteria Medica.*

Editor's Note:

Huwang Shizhe is the byname of Qianghuo, produced in the borderland in the north. It is also called Duhuo (meaning a single stem) because it stands upright. It shakes without wind and does not shake in the wind, thus called Duyao Cao (Solitary shaking grass). It is pungent and bitter in flavor, warm in property, with effects of dissipating wind caused by cold, freeing Bi syndrome (arthralgia) and relieving pain.

傳 故事

Legends and Stories

【扁鵲三兄弟】

【原文】

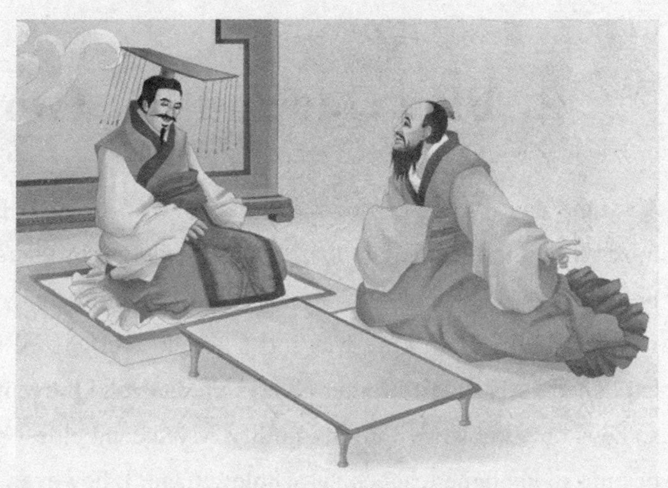

魏文王問扁鵲："子昆弟[①]三人，其孰最善爲醫？"扁鵲曰："長兄最善，中兄次之，扁鵲最爲下。"魏文王曰："可得聞邪？"扁鵲曰："長兄於病，視神未有形而除之，故名不出於家；中兄治病，其在毫毛，故名不出於閭[②]；若扁鵲者，鑱[③]血脈，投毒藥，副[④]肌膚，閒[⑤]而名出，聞於諸侯。"魏文王曰："善。"

（選自戰國・鶡冠子《鶡冠子・世賢》）

【注釋】

①昆弟：兄弟。②閭：裏巷的大門。此指鄉里。③鑱（chán 纏）：刺。④副：剖開。⑤閒（jiàn 間）：頃刻，很快。

【釋義】

有一次魏文王問扁鵲："你家兄弟三人，哪一位最精通醫術呢？"扁鵲說："大哥醫術最精，二哥次之，我最差。"魏文王問道："那爲什麼你的名氣最大呢？"扁鵲說："我大哥給人治病，是在疾病還未真正形成時就將其除掉，所以他的名氣就只在家庭范圍內；二哥治病是在疾病剛剛發生時就治愈它，所以名氣也只在附近鄉里之間；而我扁鵲治病的方法是針刺血脈、處以藥物、切開皮膚，所以名聲很快傳開，在衆多諸侯那裏也有了名氣。"魏文王說："確實是這樣啊！"

【按語】

鶡（hé 河）冠子，戰國後期的思想家，學主黄老道家，兼融諸家。生卒年不詳。其著作《鶡冠子》，過去學術界曾認爲是漢代以後的僞書，然自 1974 年長沙馬王堆帛書出土以來，學者發現《鶡冠子》有多處與帛書中的《黄帝書》意同或語同，遂確認其書作者爲鶡冠子。

本文記述的這個生動的傳説故事,借扁鵲之口形象地表達了“上工治未病”的思想。

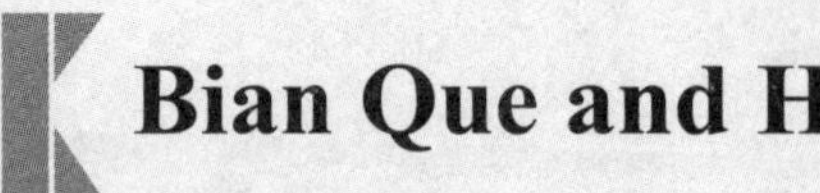

Bian Que and His Two Brothers

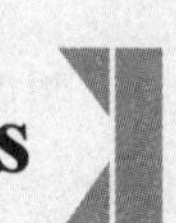

One day, King Wen of the State of Wei[1], asked Doctor Bian Que who was the most skilled in medicine among him and his two brothers. Bian Que replied, “My eldest brother is the best, my second eldest brother the second, and I rank the last.” King Wen wondered why Bian Que was most widely recognized if that was the case. Bian Que explained, “My eldest brother always predicts and prevents a disease before it breaks out, so he is only known within my family. My second eldest brother treats illness when it just occurs, so his fame reaches the whole village. I, however, cure diseases with acupuncture, medication and surgery, so many think I am a skilled doctor and my fame spread even among nobility.” King Wen agreed with this analysis.

From *Heguanzi* [2].

Notes:

1. The State of Wei (魏國) : It was a Zhou Dynasty vassal state during the Warring States Period (475–221 B.C.) of Chinese history. Its territory lay between the states of Qin and Qi and included parts of modern-day Henan, Hebei, Shanxi and Shandong. After its capital was moved from Anyi to Daliang (today Kaifeng) during the reign of King Hui of Wei, Wei was also called the State of Liang (梁國).

2. *Heguanzi* (鶡冠子 Heguanzi) : It is a book written by Heguanzi in the Warring States (475–221 B.C.).

Editor's Note:

This story vividly expressed the thought of “Preventive treatment of diseases” in traditional Chinese medicine (TCM), that is to say, a wise doctor always gives the preventive treatment before a disease occurs.

【扁鵲換心】

【原文】

魯公扈、趙齊嬰二人有疾，同請扁鵲求治。扁鵲治之既[①]同愈，謂公扈、齊嬰曰："汝曩[②]之所疾自外而干[③]府藏者，固藥石之所已[④]，今有偕生之疾[⑤]，與體偕長[⑥]，今爲汝攻之何如？"二人曰："願先聞其驗[⑦]。"扁鵲謂公扈曰："汝志强而氣弱[⑧]，故足於謀而寡於斷；齊嬰志弱而氣强[⑨]，故少於慮而傷於專。若換汝之心，則均於善矣。"扁鵲遂飲二人毒酒[⑩]，迷死[⑪]三日，剖胸探心，易而置之，投以神藥，既悟如初，二人辭歸。

于是公扈反[⑫]齊嬰之室而有其妻子，妻子弗識；齊嬰亦反公扈之室而有其妻子，妻子亦弗識。二室因相與訟[⑬]，求辨於扁鵲，扁鵲辨其所由，訟乃已。

（選自《列子 · 湯問》[⑭]）

【注釋】

①既：已經。②曩（nǎng）：從前，過去。 ③干：侵犯。 ④藥石之所已：藥物和砭石能够治好。 ⑤偕生之疾：在胎裏生的病。 ⑥偕長：謂疾病與身體共同生長。⑦其驗：指疾病的症狀和治療效果。⑧志强而氣弱：思維能力很强而缺乏勇氣。 ⑨志弱而氣强：分析思考能力很弱而膽大有勇氣。⑩毒酒：麻醉藥酒。⑪迷死：麻醉昏迷。⑫反：同"返"，下同。 ⑬訟：訴訟：即告狀。 ⑭《列子》：系東周列禦寇所作。原書早已亡佚。現存《列子》八篇，爲東晉張湛輯增。《湯問》是《列子》一書中的篇名。

【釋義】

魯國的公扈和趙國的齊嬰都生了病。同時請求扁鵲治療，都治好了。扁鵲向他兩人說："你倆過去的病，是從體外侵入内臟的，所以藥石可以治好；現在，我發現你倆有一種胎生帶來的病，跟你們的身體同時生長，我想給你倆治好怎樣？"兩人說："希望先瞭解您對這個病的診斷和治療的效果。"于是扁鵲對公扈說："你爲人很聰明，但氣質太弱，所以善於思考而缺乏决斷；齊嬰與你相反，雖然智力較差，但氣質較强，所以不善於思考，容易專横武斷。如果把你倆的心臟交换一下，那麼你們兩個人都能達到完善的地步。"扁鵲徵得兩人同意之後，便叫他倆喝了麻醉藥酒，麻醉得像死人一樣，昏迷三天没有知覺，于是剖開胸膛，拿出心臟，相互交换放置穩妥以後，用神效的藥物敷上。倆人蘇醒過來，好像正常人一樣，公扈和齊嬰便告辭，各自回家去了。

公扈回到齊嬰的家中，而親近齊嬰的妻子，但齊嬰的妻子不認識他；齊嬰也回到公扈的家，而親近公扈的妻子，公扈的妻子也不認識齊嬰。他倆的妻子都到當地官府告狀。最後，公扈、齊嬰二人請來扁鵲醫生説明真相，這兩家的官司從此才算了結。

【按語】

《列子》相傳爲戰國列禦寇所著。内容多爲民間故事、寓言和神話傳説。

《列子》記載的這一扁鵲换心的故事可謂生動形象，神乎其神。只因年代久遠，已不可確考。而中醫認爲,"心主神明""心之官則思"。《黄帝内經·素問·靈蘭秘典論》云："心者，君主之官也，神明出焉。"這則故事無疑是提供了一個佐證。將給今人以有益的啓示。

Heart Transplant Operated by Bian Que

Gong Hu from the State of Lu[1], and Qi Ying from the State of Zhao [2] were both sick. They asked Bian Que to treat them and then recovered. Afterwards, Bian Que said to them, "The disease you had was caused by external factors, and thus could be cured by medicine; but unfortunately, I found that both of you were born with a problem that is developing within the body. Shall I solve that problem for you?" The two men replied, "That's all right, but first we would like to hear your diagnosis and the treatment you propose." Bian Que said to Gong Hu, "You are intelligent, but has a weak temperament, thus are good at contemplating but poor in decision-making. On the contrary, Qi Ying lacks thoughtfulness and appears arbitrary and imperious. Therefore, the two of you would be perfect if your hearts are switched." After obtaining the two men's approval, Bian Que asked them to take some narcotic. They slept like dead men for three days. During the period, Bian Que cut open their chests, switched their hearts, and helped them heal with a special drug. They were as strong and healthy as ever when they regained consciousness.

However, because their hearts have been exchanged, Gong Hu returned to Qi Ying's home, and Qi Ying was back to Gong Hu's house. Neither man's wife and family recognize them, and the wives reported the cases to the local government. Eventually, the two men had to ask Bian Que to explain the reasons to settle the conflict.

From *Liezi* [3].

Notes:

1.The State of Lu：The State of Lu was a feudal state of the Zhou Period (1100-256 BCE). As a small state on the eastern fringe of the Central Plain, it had to cope with the ambitions of the larger states of the south and the north, especially Qi and Chu. Lu was the home state of the philosopher Confucius, and was located in the southwestern part of the modern day Shandong.

2. The State of Zhao：Zhao was one of the seven major states during the Warring States Period of ancient China. Its territory included areas in modern Inner Mongolia, Hebei, Shanxi and Shanxi Provinces. The state of Zhao bordered the Xiongnu (the Huns), the States of Qin, Wei and Yan. Its capital was Handan (邯鄲), located in modern day Hebei Province.

3. *Liezi* (《列子》Liezi)：It is a Daoist book attributed to Lie Yukou from the Warring States Period, though scholars believe that it was compiled around the 4th century BCE. The book contains numerous parables and popular stories of immortals or Daoist adepts trying to achieve longevity.

Editor's Note:

The story of Bian Que operating heart transplant was so vividly recorded in *Liezi* and it sounded miraculous. There is, however, no way to know if this had happened for sure because it was so long ago. In TCM, heart is regarded as "the monarch of all the organs." This story provides a strong evidence of the functions of the heart.

【橘井】

【原文】

蘇耽[1]，桂陽[2]人也，漢文帝[3]時得道，人稱蘇仙。公早喪所怙[4]，鄉里以仁孝著聞，宅在郡城東北，距縣治百餘里。公與母共食，母曰："無鮓[5]。"公即輟筯[6]，起身取錢而去。須臾以鮓至。母曰："何所得來？"公曰："縣市。"母曰："去縣道往返百餘里，頃刻而至，汝欺我也！"公曰："買鮓時，見舅氏，約明日至。"次日，舅果至。一日，雲間儀衛降宅[7]。公語母曰："某受命仙籙[8]，當違色養[9]。"母曰："我何存活？"公以兩盤留。母需飲食，扣小盤，需錢帛扣大盤，所需皆立至。

又語母曰："明年天下疾疫，庭中井水橘樹能療。患疫者，與井水一升，橘葉一枚，飲之立愈。"後果然，求水葉者，遠至千里，應手而愈。

（選自漢 · 劉向《列仙傳》⑩）

【注釋】

①蘇耽（dān 丹）：西漢文帝時期人。後人譽爲神仙。②桂陽：郡名，今湖南省郴州市一帶。③漢文帝：漢高祖劉邦之子，名劉恒，前179—前157年在位。④早喪所怙（hù 户）：早年死了父親。⑤鮓（zhǎ 眨）：指經過腌制的魚類食品。⑥輟筯（chuò zhù 綽住）：放下筷子。⑦雲間儀衛降宅：天上的儀仗隊從空中降落蘇氏住宅。⑧某受命仙籙：我接受了上天的命令，名字已載入神仙簿籍。籙，簿籍，記載天上官吏姓名的素書。⑨當違色養：必將離開家庭，不能奉養老人而盡孝了。色養，舊時泛稱盡孝。⑩劉向（前77—前6）：名更生，字子政，今江蘇徐州人，漢皇族楚元王劉交之四世孫。曾主持校閱群書，撰成目録書《别録》，另有《新序》《説苑》《列女傳》等。《列仙傳》：二卷，舊題漢劉向撰，系後人僞托，實爲東漢人所作。内容記載神仙故事七十則。

【釋義】

蘇耽，湖南郴州人，在西漢文帝時期，他懂得了養生之道，人們稱他爲蘇仙。蘇耽早年喪父，周圍鄉里都知道他是孝敬母親的人。他家住在縣城東北，離城一百餘里。有一次，蘇耽與母親正吃飯間，母親對他說，"没有腌魚呀！"蘇耽立即放下筷子，起身取錢走出門去，不一會就拿着腌魚回來。母親驚奇地問他："從哪裏買來的？"蘇耽說："從縣城裏買的。"母親說："自家到縣城往返一百餘里，這麼一會兒就回來，你在欺騙我呀！"蘇耽對母親說："我買魚的時候，遇見舅舅，與舅約定，明天到咱家來。"第二天，蘇耽的舅舅果然到來。

有一天，天上的儀仗隊降落蘇宅。蘇耽對母親說："我已受命爲天上的仙人了，今天就要離開人間，再不能奉養母親了。"蘇耽的母親說，"那我怎麼活下去呢？"蘇耽留下兩個盤子，母親需要飲食就敲小盤子，需要錢財和布帛就敲大盤子，所要的東西都能立即送到。

蘇耽又對母親說："明年天下發生流行疫病，院子裏的井水和橘樹能够治療。如有患病的人，給他一升井水，一片橘葉，煎湯飲服，立可痊愈。"後來果然發生疫病，遠至千里之遥的人，都來求井水橘葉，凡是飲了井水橘葉的病人，其病便立即痊愈。

【按語】

托名劉向所著的《列仙傳》，是一部記載列位元神仙形跡的著作。所述事跡，幾乎皆與長生仙去、神通變化諸方術有關，反映出兩漢時期神仙方士的活躍情況。爲後世道教神仙故事的重要來源之一。尤其黄帝等故事，多被引用。

劉向（約前77—前6），原名更生，字子政，祖籍沛郡（今屬江蘇徐州）。西漢著名學者。漢成帝時擔任光禄大夫，曾全面主持各類書籍的整理校勘工作，成果甚豐。所撰《别録》，爲中國目録學之祖。

關於《列仙傳》的著作朝代和撰人，歷來聚訟頗多，但一般認爲，並非西漢劉向所撰。有的疑爲東漢之作，《四庫提要》認爲是魏晉間文士所爲。本文記述的是仙人蘇耽的故事。正是由於這位仙人蘇耽告知“庭中井水橘樹能療病”，後又果然應驗，于是便形成了“橘井”這一典故。所謂“橘井泉香”“龍蟠橘井”等語，皆源於此。如今，郴州市内尚有橘井，是後人爲紀念蘇耽所建。

The Orange Tree and the Well

Su Dan was born in Chenzhou, Hunan Province. He became a great master in life-nurturing techniques and was recognized as an immortal during the period of Emperor Wen of Han (202–157 BCE). His father died when Su was young. He showed dedication and filial piety to his mother. One day, his mother said on the dining table that they have run out of smoked fish. He immediately put his chopsticks down, took some money and went out. Minutes later, he came back with smoked fish. His mother said in surprise, “Where did you get it?” He replied, “I bought it from the town.” She could not believe it, saying, “It’s over 100 Li from our home to the town, how can you return home so soon? You must be lying to me!” He explained, “On my way I run into my uncle and asked him to come here tomorrow.” On the next day, his uncle did come.

One day, messengers from the heaven descended at his home. Su said to his mother, “My name has entered the register of immortals. I feel a great pity that I have to leave you now and will never have the opportunity to look after you.” She said, “How can I survive without you?" Su told her that he would leave two dishes and she may clink the smaller one for food, and the bigger one for money or cloth. The things she desired would be sent in no time.

After that, he told his mother that an epidemic would break out the next year, and the well and the orange tree in their yard can provide the cure. By boiling a leaf in a sheng of well water, any patient will recover at once. The next year, the epidemic spread just as Su had predicted. Patients, even those from thousands of Li away, came to seek for help and were cured instantly.

From *Biographies of Immortals* [1].

Notes:

1. *Biographies of Immortals* (《列仙傳》Liexian Zhuan): It is a book written by Liu Xiang in the Han Dynasty (206 BCE–220).

Editor's Note:

Biographies of Immortals is one of the important sources of legends and Daoist ways of life nurturing for later generations.

【彭祖長壽】

【原文】

彭祖,姓籛(jiān 笺),諱①鏗,帝顓頊②之玄孫也。殷末已七百六十七歲,而不衰老。王令采女乘輜軿③,往問道於彭祖。彭祖曰:"吾遺腹④而生,三歲而失母,遇犬戎⑤之亂,流離西域,百有餘年。加以少枯⑥,失四十九妻,喪五十四子,數遭憂患,和氣⑦折傷,榮衛焦枯,恐不度世⑧。所聞淺薄,不足宣傳。"乃去,不知所之。其後七十餘年,聞人於流沙之國西見之。

(選自晉 · 葛洪《神仙傳》卷一)

【注釋】

①諱:古代死者之名叫諱。②顓頊(zhuān xū 専虚):古帝名,五帝之一。相傳

爲黄帝之孫,號高陽氏。③采女:從民間采擇進宫廷供役使的少女,即宫女。輜軿(zī píng 資平):古時貴族乘坐的一種有帷蓋的車子。④遺腹:指父已死而子始生。⑤犬戎:古時西方的一個民族。⑥少枯:指年少時身體弱。⑦和氣:中和之氣。⑧不度世:不久于人世。

【釋義】

彭祖，姓籛，名鏗，所以又叫他彭鏗，是顓頊帝的玄孫。殷代末年，他已活了七百六十七歲，外貌却不顯得衰老。殷王羡慕彭祖長壽，便派遣宫女坐了輜軿車向彭祖請問長生之道。彭祖説："我是遺腹生的兒子，媽媽撫養我到三歲，也死了。剩下我這個孤兒，後來又遭遇到北方犬戎的禍亂，流離到西域，過了一百多年。我年少的時候，身體本來不大結實，活到現在，總共死去四十九個妻子，喪亡了五十四個兒子，數次經歷人生憂患，精神上受到很大影響，營衛氣血都已焦枯，恐怕不久於人世了。我所知道的養生之道，實在淺薄得很，哪裏值得宣揚啊！"於是悄悄離去，不知到了什麽地方。這以後又過了七十多年，纔聽人説曾在流沙國以西見過他。

【按語】

由晉代葛洪所撰《神仙傳》，是道教神仙信仰的书籍之一。

葛洪的《神仙傳》一書,收録了古代傳説中的九十二位仙人的神奇故事。旨在宣揚"神仙可學，不死可得"的思想，顯然是荒誕的，但其中的一些醫學文獻和道家的養生方法，倒有不少可取之處。而書中塑造的一系列仙人形象,也爲後世的小説創作提供了素材。

彭祖長壽的神話傳説,在戰國時代就有流傳了。《楚辭·天問》説:"彭鏗斟雉帝何饗?受壽永多夫何悵?"意思是彭鏗斟了他親自烹調的野鷄湯奉獻給天帝，天帝吃了滿心歡喜，賜給了他那麽長的壽命，臨死時他爲什麽還要感到惆悵？看來是天帝賜給了彭祖長壽的生命，使彭祖一直活到八百餘歲。而有趣的是彭祖並不滿足，仍嫌身體不够健康，還想由長壽達到永生不死。這就使後世的道家方士們得以在彭祖身上塗抹上許多仙話的色彩。

Peng Zu's Secret for Longevity

Peng Zu, the great-great-grandson of Emperor Zhuan Xu[1], was also named Peng Keng. Although he had been 767 years old by the end of the Yin Dynasty (ca. 1600 BCE–1200 BCE), he did not appear aged at all. The King of Yin envied his longevity and sent a lady-in-waiting to ask his secret method. Peng Zu replied, "My father died before I was born, and my mother passed away when I reached the age of three. I was left all alone. Following the revolt caused by the nomads from the north, I had to flee to the western part of the country for over a hundred years. I was not in good health when I was young. During my life, I survived my 49 wives and 54 sons, and experienced endless sufferings. All these combined had left me in poor shape. I am afraid that I will not be around that much longer. The knowledge that I acquired about life nurturing is too superficial to share. " Therefore, he left unnoticed, with no one knowing his whereabouts. It was not until about 70 years later that he was reportedly seen in the western area bordering the Liusha Country.

From *Biographies of Divine Immortals*.

Notes:

1. Emperor Zhuan Xu: Zhuan Xu was a mythological emperor of ancient China. He was the grandson of the Yellow Emperor (2698 BCE–2598 BCE).

Editor's Note:

Compiled by the Daoist scholar and polymath Ge Hong, the book *Biographies of Divine Immortals* included fantasy stories of 92 so-called immortals. These stories were to promote the techniques of long-living and life nurturing, which, if done properly, was said to lead to immortality. As absurd as the idea of immortality was, the book suggested some principles and methods that were beneficial to human health.

【杏林】

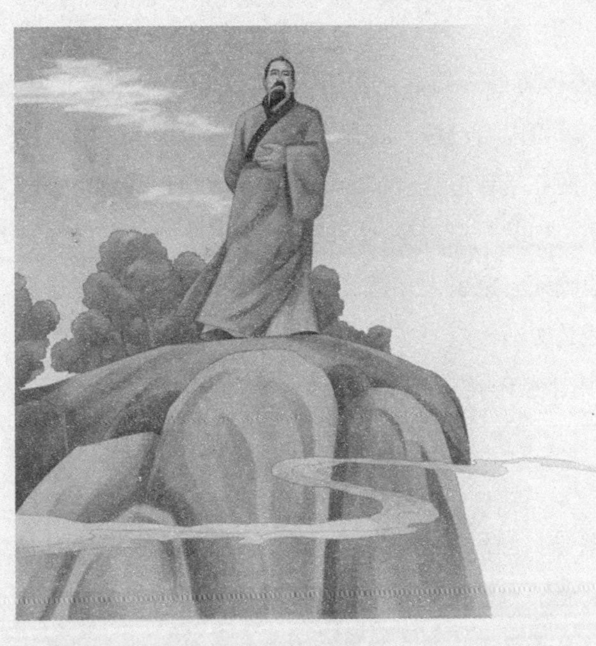

【原文】

董奉[①]者，字君異，侯官[②]人也……後還豫章[③]，廬山[④]下居。……奉居山不種田，日爲人治病，亦不取錢。重病愈者，使栽杏五株，輕者一株，如此數年，得十萬餘株，鬱然[⑤]成林。乃使山中百禽群獸游戲其下，卒不生草，常如芸治[⑥]也。

後杏子大熟，于林中作一草倉，示時人曰：欲買杏者，不須報奉，但將穀一器置倉中，即自往取一器杏去。嘗有人置穀少而取杏去多者，林中群虎出吼逐之，大怖[⑦]，急挈杏走路旁，傾覆。至家量杏，一如穀多少。或有人偷杏者，虎逐之到家，嚙[⑧]至死。家人知其偷杏，乃送還奉，叩頭謝過，乃却[⑨]使活。奉每年貨杏得穀，旋以賑救貧乏，供給行旅不逮者[⑩]，歲二萬餘人。

（選自晉 · 葛洪《神仙傳》[⑪]）

【注釋】

①董奉：三國時期吳國的民間醫生。②侯官：舊縣名，西漢置，治所在今福州市。③豫章：郡名，楚漢置。今南昌市。④廬山：一名匡廬，在江西省九江市南部。⑤鬱然：繁盛的樣子。⑥芸治：鋤耕管理。⑦怖：惶懼的樣子。⑧嚙（niè 聶）：咬。⑨却：又。⑩行旅不逮者：外出旅行經濟困難、物資不能供應的人。⑪葛洪（281—341）：字稚川，自號抱朴子，丹陽句容（今江蘇句容）人，東晉醫藥學家、道家。著有《神仙傳》《抱朴子》《肘後方》等。《神仙傳》敘述了九十二位神仙的故事。

【釋義】

董奉，字君異，東吳侯官人。……後來回到南昌，就在廬山定居下來。……董奉住在山上而不種地，每天爲人治病，不取分文。如果重病治好了，讓病人栽五棵杏樹；輕病治好了，栽一棵杏樹。這樣連續好些年，所種的杏樹已有十萬餘棵，鬱鬱葱葱，茂密成林，因而使得山中的各種飛禽走獸都游戲在杏林之中，一年到頭不長雜草，像經常耕鋤管理過一樣。

後來，杏子大量成熟，董奉就在杏林裏搭一糧倉，告訴人們：有買杏子的人，不必告訴我，只將容器的穀子倒入糧倉，就可以自己取一容器杏子走。曾有一人，放入的穀子少而取走的杏子多，杏林裏的老虎便怒吼着追趕。那人十分害怕，急忙提着杏子順路旁逃跑，不料跌倒在地，杏子撒了許多。到家一量杏子，竟和送去的穀子一樣多。有時，有偷杏子的人，老虎就追他到家，把他咬死。家裏人知道後，就把偷來的杏子照數送還董奉，叩頭賠禮認錯，于是董奉竟又使其復活。

董奉每年用杏換得穀子，隨後又用來救濟周圍的貧苦百姓，接濟來盧山旅行而斷了盤費的人，每年救濟約有二萬多人。

【按語】

這個故事雖有神話色彩，但董奉居山，“日爲人治病，亦不取錢”的事迹，至今仍傳爲美談。“杏林”美名滿天下，漸漸地成了“醫林”的代名詞。廣大醫家偏愛“杏林”，以杏自喻，以杏自號，以杏爲書名，以杏爲頌語。病人贈送給醫生的匾額，常書“杏林春暖”“譽滿杏林”“功滿杏林”等。對聯中常有“虎守杏林春日暖，龍蟠橘井水泉香”“董氏杏林憑虎守，蘇家橘井有龍蟠”（見“橘井”條）等佳句。“杏林”二字，也常爲醫藥團體、刊物、賓館所使用，如“杏林學社”“杏林叢録”“杏林賓館”等。日本也有“漢方杏林會”等。其實，人們愛“杏林”，正是愛的“救死扶傷”“施藥濟貧”的杏林精神。這種精神正是中華民族的傳統之光。

The Apricot Orchard

Dong Feng, whose style name is Jun Yi, was born in Houguan County during the Three Kingdoms Period. He settled in Lushan Mountain area but did not farm. Day after day he treated patients without any charge. Whenever he rescued a patient from a severe disease, he would ask the patient to plant five apricot trees, for a minor illness, one apricot tree. Within several years, more than one hundred thousand apricot trees were planted and formed a gigantic and exuberant orchard, with numerous birds and beasts living in it. Wild grass did not grow there as if someone meticulously maintained it.

When all the apricots were ripe, he built a granary in the orchard and told the local people to put some grains in the granary if they wanted the same amount of apricot, and they did not have to notify him. And people did. Those who gave less than they took would always be identified and chased by the tigers living in the orchard. There was such a person, who took more than he deserved, so the tigers came out. The man was terrified and tried to run, but he fell down on the way and lost many apricots. When he got home, he weighed the apricots, only to find that what was left was the exact amount he should have taken. There were occasions when the tigers followed those who stole the apricots and killed them. Their family members would then return the apricots and kneel down to plea for forgiveness. Dong Feng would bring the deceased people back to life.

Every year, Dong Feng exchanged apricots for grains, which he used to relieve the starved and those who ran out of supplies when traveled to the Lushan Mountain. His good will benefited more than 20,000 people every year.

From *Biographies of Divine Immortals*.

Editor's Note:

In this excerpt, Doctor Dong Feng asked his patients to plant apricot trees instead of paying medical fees. From then on, "apricot orchard" became a euphemism for the medical profession. Many doctors and common people favored this term, and it is often used to name journals, medical organizations and hotels. People love this word because they love the spirit to heal the wounded and rescue the dying. This is the true spirit of the TCM tradition.

松脂愈癩

【原文】

聞上黨[①]有趙瞿者，病癩歷年，衆治之不愈，垂死。或云不如及活流棄[②]之，後子孫轉相注易[③]，其家乃賫糧，將之送置山穴中。瞿在穴中，自怨不幸，晝夜悲嘆，涕泣經月。有仙人行經過穴，見而哀之，具問訊之。瞿知其異人，乃叩頭自陳乞哀，于是仙人以一囊藥賜之，教其服法。瞿服之百許日，瘡都愈，顏色丰悅，肌膚玉澤。仙人又過視之，瞿謝受更生活[④]之恩，乞丐[⑤]其方。仙人告之曰："此是松脂耳，此山中更多此物，汝煉之，服，可以長生不死。"瞿乃歸家。家人初謂之鬼也，甚驚愕。瞿遂長服松脂，身體轉輕，氣力百倍，登危越險，終日不極[⑥]。年百七十歲，齒不墮，髮不白。

（選自晉・葛洪《抱朴子内篇》卷十一）

【注釋】

①上黨：地名，在今山西長治市。②流棄：流徙抛棄。③注易：這裏指流動轉易。④更生活：又獲得再生。⑤丐：給予。⑥極：疲倦。

【釋義】

聽説上黨有個叫趙瞿的，得了癩病好幾年，衆多醫生都治不好，快要死了。有人説，不如趁他活着時就流徙抛棄他。後來子孫們相互流動轉易，他的家人又帶着糧食，抬着他，把他送到山洞中。趙瞿在洞中，埋怨自己的不幸，晝夜悲嘆，哭了好幾個月。有個仙人行游經過山洞，看見了他，感到可憐，一一訊問他。趙瞿知道這是個奇異的人，就叩頭自述，乞求憐憫。于是仙人拿一袋藥賞賜給他，教給他服食的方法。趙瞿服用藥一百多天，瘡疤都長好了，顏面丰滿神色愉悦，肌膚潤澤。仙人又經過看視他。趙瞿道謝使自己獲得再生的恩德，乞求這種藥方。仙人告訴他説："這不過是松脂而已。這座山中有很多這種藥物，你熔煉後服用，可以因此而長生不死。"趙瞿回到家，家裏人開始認爲他是個鬼，非常驚愕。趙瞿從此後長期服食松脂，身體變得更輕，力氣增加百倍，登上高嶺，翻越險峰，整天不覺累。享年一百七十歲，牙齒不落，頭髮不白。

【按語】

《抱朴子内篇》是晉代葛洪的著作，为现存体系最完整的"神仙家言"，对道教理论有一定的发展。

松脂，又稱松香、松膏、松肪、松膠香等。松脂爲松樹油脂所提制，因其脂通明，宛如熏陸香，所以又稱松香，古代養生家常煉之服食，不過它更多的是應用於外科。其性味苦、甘、温，有燥濕、殺蟲、止癢、拔毒、生肌之功效，故多塗擦瘡疥濕瘡，用於癰疽癤疔。

本文講述了服食松脂的神奇功效，未免有傳説的成分。

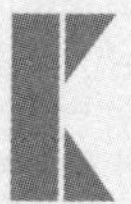

Pine Resin, the Cure for Leprosy

It was said that there was a man named Zhao Qu from Changzhi City of Shanxi Province who had suffered from leprosy. He was dying from this incurable disease. Some suggested he be abandoned despite he was still alive. None of his children or grandchildren was willing to take care of him, and eventually his family brought him to a cave and left him there with some food. Sighing and weeping, Zhao stayed in the cave and lamented all day and night for his misfortune. One day, an immortal happened to pass the cave and found him there. He pitied Zhao and asked why he was so sad. Zhao knew that this man must be extraordinary, and so he knelt down and begged for sympathy. The immortal thus handed him a bag of medicine and taught him how to take it.

After taking the medicine for more than one hundred days, Zhao completely recovered, with smooth skin and fine complexion. When the immortal visited him again, Zhao thanked him repeatedly and asked about the magical formula. The immortal told him that it was nothing but pine resin, which was abundant in the mountain. After melting it, one can take it and achieve longevity.

Zhao went back home and shocked his family, who at first thought he was a ghost. Zhao's strength was now doubled and he became more flexible ever since he started to take the resin every day. He did not feel tired at all even after climbing mountains or traveling a long way. His teeth and hair remained when he passed away at the age of 170.

From *The Instrinsic Aspect of Embraces Simplicity* [1].

Notes:

1. *The Instrinsic Aspect of Embraces Simplicity* (《抱朴子内篇》 Baopuzi Neipian): It is an important Daoist text written by Ge Hong (葛洪 284-364) in the Eastern Jin Dynasty (東晉 317-420).

Editor's Note:

Pine resin, also known as turpentine, is extracted and refined from pine oil. It looks transparent like pistacia lentiscus and is often applied to surgery. It is bitter sweet and warm in nature. It can reduce dampness within the human body, relieve itching, detoxify the body and promote tissue growth. It is often used to treat scabies, carbuncle, gangrene, furuncle and malignant boil. With a touch of fantasy, this excerpt tells the magic effects of pine resin.

【懸壺】

【原文】

市中有一老翁，懸一壺於肆頭①。及市罷，輒跳入壺中。市人莫之見，惟長房②於樓上睹之，異焉。因往再拜，奉酒脯③；翁知長房之意其神④也，謂之曰："子明日可更來。"長房旦日復詣翁，翁乃與俱入壺中。惟見玉堂嚴麗⑤，旨酒甘肴⑥，盈衍⑦其中。共飲畢而出。後長房欲求道，隨從入山。翁撫之曰："子可教也。"遂能醫療衆病……

（選自南朝 · 范曄⑧《後漢書》）

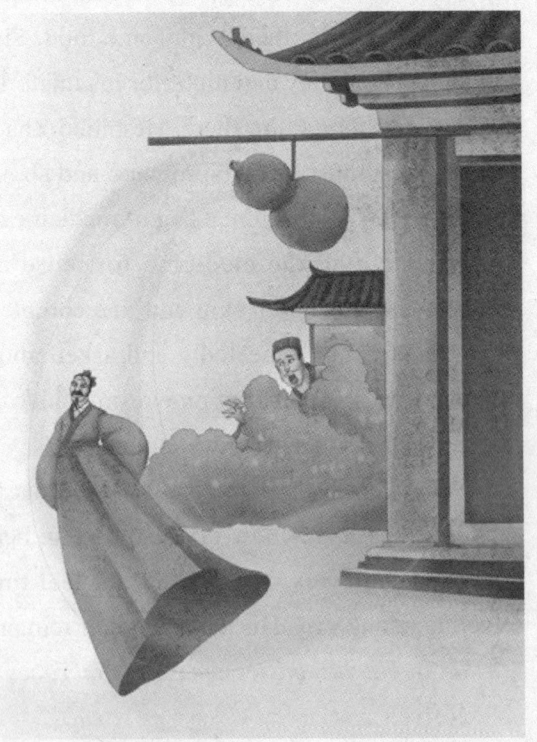

【注釋】

①肆頭：店鋪門首。 ②長房：即費長房，東漢時期的巫醫，汝南（今河南省汝南縣）人。曾爲市掾（yuàn 院），即管理集市場所的小官。③脯（fǔ 府）：乾肉。④意其神：認爲他是神人。⑤玉堂嚴麗：殿堂莊嚴華麗。玉堂，亦指神仙居處。⑥旨

酒甘肴：美好的酒肉食物。⑦盈衍：充滿。⑧范曄（yè 葉，398—445）：南朝宋史學家，字蔚宗，順陽（今河南淅川東）人。綜合各家之長而撰《後漢書》，它記載了上起漢光武帝、下至漢獻帝一百九十六年的歷史。

【釋義】

集市之中有一老翁賣藥，他在店鋪門前懸掛着一個大空壺，等到集市散去，總是跳入壺中。集上的人都没有看見過他，只有管理市場的小官費長房在樓上看到此事，感到非常驚奇。于是其前去拜望老翁，並送給他美好的酒肉食物。老翁知道費長房認爲他是一位神人，便對費長房説："您明天可以再來。"第二天，費長房又去拜望老翁，老翁便邀他同入壺中。費長房只見宫廷華麗莊嚴，美酒佳餚滿桌，二人暢飲盡興而出。後來，費長房願向老翁學習醫道，便跟老翁隱居山中。老翁欣慰地撫摸着費長房説："您求學心誠，我願意把醫道方術傳授給您。"後來，費長房終於把老翁的醫術繼承下來，在民間爲廣大群衆治病……

【按語】

"懸壺"這一典故，晉·葛洪《神仙傳》中亦有類似的記載，只是鬼神味濃一些。其文曰："壺公者，不知其姓名也。……時費長房見公從遠方來，入市賣藥，人莫之識，賣藥不二價，治病皆愈。每語人曰："服此藥必吐某物，某日當愈。"言無不效。常懸一空壺於屋上，日入跳入壺中。長房知非常人，乃日掃公座前地，及供饌物，公受不辭。積久，長房不少懈，亦不敢有求。公知長房篤信，謂曰，"暮更來。"長房如其言，公爲傳封符一卷，付之曰："帶此可主諸鬼神常稱使者，可以治病消災。"長房乃行符收鬼，治病無不愈者。

後世醫生開業，常以"懸壺"稱之。醫生治病救人，稱爲"懸壺濟世"。"懸壺"一詞，即來源於此。

The Hanging Pot

There was once an elder selling medicine in a market, with an empty pot hanging in front of his store. Every time the market closed, he would jump into the pot. Nobody noticed it except Fei Zhangfang, a low-ranking official managing the market. He found it unbelievable, so he paid the elder a visit and invited him for a nice meal. Knowing that Fei thought he was a divine being, the elder invited Fei to come along into the pot tomorrow.

The next day, Fei visited the elder and both went in the pot. Fei was amazed by the magnificent palace as well as superb food and drinks he found in the pot. They fully enjoyed the feast. Later, Fei expressed his wish to retreat into the mountain with the elder to learn medicine. The elder gladly patted him on the back, saying, "Since you are sincere to learn medicine, it would be my pleasure to teach you all I know." Fei then became knowledgeable and skilled in medicine, and saved the lives of many and relieved the pain for more.

From *The Book of the Later Han Dynasty* [1].

Notes:

1. *The Book of the Later Han Dynasty* (《後漢書》Houhanshu): A historical text produced with official sponsorship, covering the history of the Later Han Dynasty from 6 to 189. It was compiled by Fan Ye and others in the fifth century during the Liu Song Dynasty, using a number of earlier histories and documents as sources.

Editor's Note:

The book *Biographies of Divine Immortals* (《神仙傳》Shenxianzhuan) by Ge Hong also has a similar record about the story "the Hanging Pot" , but even more absurd from the modern perspective. Because of this legend, people often said "hanging pot" when doctors started to practice medicine. Thus, the idiom "Hanging pot to relieve the sufferings in this world" means to cure illnesses and save human lives.

【偓佺食松子】

【原文】

偓佺[①]者,槐山采藥父也,好食松實。形體生毛,長七寸,兩目更方。能飛行,逐走馬。以松子遺[②]堯,堯不暇服。松者,簡松[③]也。時受服者,皆三百歲。

(選自晉 · 干寶《搜神記 · 偓佺》)

【注釋】

①偓(wò 握)佺:傳説中古仙人名。《史記 · 司馬相如傳》有"偓佺之倫暴于南榮"之語。意思是説偓佺這些神仙在南邊的屋檐下曬太陽。《列仙傳》中也記載了他的故事,内容和《搜神記》基本相同。尚有"遺贈堯門,貽此神方"等句,意思是秘術送給堯帝,留下長壽秘方。 ②遺(wèi 畏):贈予。 ③簡松:大松。

【釋義】

偓佺是槐山的采藥老人,他喜歡吃松樹的果實。身體上長着七寸長的毛,雙眼變成了方形,能奔走如飛,追趕那奔跑着的馬。他曾將松子贈送給堯,堯没有閑置時間服用。這種松樹,都是大松,當時所服用的松樹子,都已長了三百年了。

【按語】

若説食松子能成仙,當然是無稽之談,但松子確實對人體有益。陶弘景《名醫别録》列之上品。李時珍在《本草綱目》中説:松子"氣味甘,小温,無毒"。並引用《開寶本草》等書説:"逐風痹寒氣,虚羸少氣,補不足,潤皮膚,肥五臟。主諸風,温腸胃。久服,輕身延年不老。"還特意引述了偓佺食松子的故事。據現代藥理實驗研究,松子含有多種氨基酸和維生素,具有增强免疫、抗衰老的功能。看來,當把松子視作養生之品。

Wo Quan Ate Pine Nuts

Wo Quan, an old man gathering medicinal herbs in Huaishan Mountain, was fond of pine nuts. Truly an unusual being, he grew hair on his body as long as seven inches, and his eyes were square-shaped. He could run as fast as if he was flying, and was able to catch up with running horses. He once offered the pine nuts to King Yao, one of the great rulers from China's legendary period of antiquity. However, Yao was too busy to take it. Those pine trees were all very big, which had been around for 300 years.

From *Anecdotes about Spirits and Immortals* [1].

Note:

1. *Anecdotes about Spirits and Immortals* (《搜神記》Soushenji): This novel was written during the dynasties of Wei and Jin. The author Gan Bao recorded a number of legends and unusual stories about humans and other beings and shed light on the spiritual world of the Chinese at that time.

Editor's Note:

It is absurd to maintain that people who eat pine nuts can become immortal, and pine nuts are indeed beneficial to the human body. As Li Shizhen put in his *Compendium of Materia Medica*, pine nuts are "sweet, slightly warm in nature and non-toxic". According to modern pharmacological studies, pine nuts contain a variety of amino acids and vitamins and can enhance immunity and delay the aging process. It is good for maintaining health.

【梵僧吹鼻治息肉】

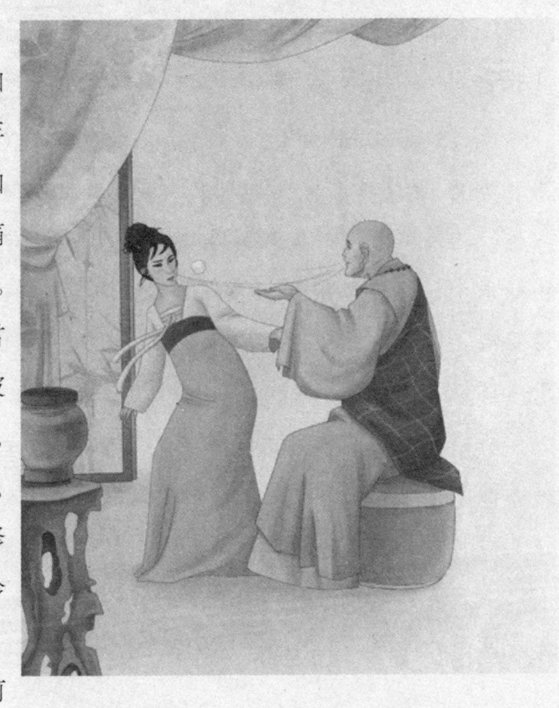

【原文】

永貞[①]年，東市百姓[②]王布，知書，藏鏹[③]千萬，高旅多賓之[④]。有女年十四五，豔麗聰悟，鼻兩孔各垂息肉如皂莢子，其根如麻綫，長寸許，觸之痛入心髓。其父破錢數百萬治之，不瘥。忽一日，有梵僧[⑤]乞食，因問布："知君女有異疾，可一見，吾能止之。"布被問大喜。即見其女，僧乃取藥，色正白，吹其鼻中。少頃，摘去之。出少黄水，都無所苦。布賞之百金，梵僧曰："吾修道之人，不受厚施，唯乞此息肉。"遂珍重而去，行疾如飛，布亦意其賢聖也。

（選自唐・段成式《酉陽雜俎》前集卷一）

【注釋】

①永貞：唐順宗李誦年號，指805年，年號永貞。 ②百姓：古代對貴族的總稱。③鏹（qiǎng 搶）：錢串，引申爲成串的錢。 ④賓之：把他當賓客看待。賓，意動用法。⑤梵（fàn 范）僧：印度僧人。也稱佛僧。梵語爲古印度書面語，故對印度等地的事物，常冠以梵字。又佛經原用梵語寫成，故凡與佛有關的事物，皆稱梵。

【釋義】

唐代永貞年間，長安東市場一貴族王布，頗有學問，家藏有千萬串的錢，富商大賈多把他當賓客對待。他有個女兒，年齡十四五歲，生得艷麗聰慧；可是，兩個鼻孔各垂下一塊如皂莢子大的息肉。息肉的根細如麻綫，長一寸多，若觸動它，疼痛鑽心入髓。她父親花錢數百萬進行治療，均無效果。忽然有一天，有一佛僧來求食，於是問王布："聞知您女兒有奇疾，可否讓見一見，我能治療這種病。"王布被詢問，非常高興。立即讓女兒來見，和尚於是取出白色藥面，吹入病人鼻孔。一會兒工夫，就摘掉了息肉，流出少量黄水，但病人始終没有感到痛苦。王布拿出百兩黄金賞他，和尚説："我是修道之人，不接受豐厚的布施，只要這兩塊息肉就行了。"於是，小心地包好息肉就離去，行走快如飛。王布覺得他大概是一位聖賢之人。

【按語】

段成式（803—863），字柯古，晚唐鄒平（今山東鄒平縣）人，後遷居臨淄（今山東淄博）。唐代著名志怪小説家、藏書家。在詩壇上，他與李商隱、温庭筠齊名。因三人排行均爲第十六，故時號"三十六體"。他曾任江州刺史，因事被罷官。後游弋於青山緑水中，終日以讀書、著書自娱，以藏書、校書爲事。他能詩善文，除代表作《酉陽雜俎》傳世外，在《全唐詩》中還收入他的詩三十多首，《全唐文》中收入他的文章十一篇。

所著志怪小説集《酉陽雜俎》二十卷，《續集》十卷，以内容廣博而蜚聲中外。凡神道仙佛、天文地理、文化藝術、風俗民情、動植貨殖、奇聞逸事，幾乎無所不載。保存了南北朝至唐代的許多珍貴史料，對後世的文學創作産生了較大影響。

本文這則故事，有神話色彩，不必究其真。而那位佛僧不計回報施醫舍藥的美德，却是值得發揚的。

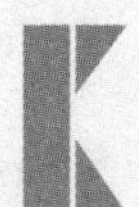

A Monk from Afar Removed Polyps

During the Yongzhen years of the Tang Dynasty (618-907), Wang Bu, a noble man living on the west side of Chang'an, was well-learned and wealthy, so much so that other rich people treated him as a truly distinguished individual. His daughter was about 14 or 15 years old, and was really beautiful and smart. Unfortunately, she suffered from two sizable polyps dropping from her nostrils. The roots of the polyps, as thin as strings, were about 3 centimeters long. A touch of the polyp would cause her stabbing pain. Wang had spent millions on finding a cure for his daughter but all his efforts were in vain.

One day, a Buddhist monk came to beg for food. Then he said, "I heard that your daughter has got a rare disease. Would you like me to have a look to see if I could find a cure for her?" Wang Bu was beyond delight and sent for his daughter immediately. The monk blew some white medicinal powder into her nostrils. After a while, the polyps fell with some yellowish pus discharged from her noses, but it did not cause her any pain. Wang Bu prepared lots of gold to thank the monk, but he declined the generosity, saying, "I'm just a monk and I want to take nothing but these polyps." Having obtained the permission, he wrapped the polyps with great care and left, moving swiftly as if he had wings. Wang Bu thought that he must be an extraordinary being.

From *Miscellaneous Records by Duan Chengshi*[1].

Notes:

1. *Miscellaneous Records by Duan Chengshi* (《酉陽雜俎》Youyang Zazu): is a collection of writings on mythical creatures, unusual incidents, anecdotes and legends. Written by Duan Chengshi who lived in the Late Tang Dynasty, it was a fine reference book for studying literature, history, natural science, and other subjects of that time. It has been widely quoted and canonized by famous writers and scholars in later generations.

【滴芝難得】

【原文】

少室石户①中，更有深谷，不可得過。以石投谷中，半日猶聞其聲也。去户外十餘丈，有石柱，柱上有偃蓋石②，南度徑可一丈許③。望之，蜜芝從石上隨石偃蓋中，良久，輒有一滴。有似雨屋後之餘漏，時時一落耳。然蜜芝墮不息，而偃蓋亦終滴也。户上刻石爲科斗字④，曰："得服石蜜芝一斗者，壽萬歲。"諸道士共思惟其處，不可得往。唯當以碗器置勁竹木端，以承取之。然竟⑤未有能爲之者。按此户上刻題如此，前世必已有之者也。

（選自《太平廣記 · 草木》）

【注釋】

①少室石户：嵩山少室山的石洞。②偃蓋石：仰卧若蓋的石頭。③"南度"句：向南伸出估計有一丈左右的方圓。④科斗：同蝌蚪。漢字字體之一，即科斗篆，據説爲倉頡所造。⑤竟：最終。

【釋義】

嵩山少室山的石洞中，又有深谷，不能通過。以石投谷中，老半天纔能聽到其聲音。距離洞外十餘丈，有根石柱。柱上有仰卧若蓋的石頭，向南伸出估計有一丈左右的方圓。向上望，蜜芝從石上順着石偃蓋往下流，好大一會兒，纔有一滴。就像下雨屋後的餘漏，不斷地往下落。然而蜜芝落不止，也就始終順着偃蓋石往下滴。洞口石上刻有蝌蚪文字，説："能服石蜜芝一斗的人，壽命可達一萬歲。"衆道士都想着石洞那個地方，可是不能上去。只能用碗一類器物置放在堅勁的竹木頂端，用來承取之。然而始終没有誰能做到。按説此洞上有如此的刻石，前世必定已有人上去了。

【按語】

説"服石蜜芝一斗，壽命可達一萬歲"，未免是誇張之辭。正是因爲它珍貴，才使衆多的人嚮往之，然而始終没有誰能得到。只有望山而興嘆。看來這種長生不死的神藥是難以得到的。

The Unattainable Honey Drip

There was a stone cave in the Shaoshi ridge of the Songshan Mountain. It was impossible to access because of a wide and deep valley. If one threw a stone into the valley, the echo would last for a long while. Dozens of meters away from the cave, there stood a stone pillar. A rock sat on top of the pillar, reaching out for about 3 meters. Looking up, one could see honey dripping from the rock, and the echo of each drip could be heard a few moments later.

The honey kept dripping, just like rainwater permeating a roof, day and night. Carved on the stove cave were characters of an ancient script style, which read, "Those who can drink 1 dou (斗，a unit of dry measure for grain，equivalently 1 decalitre) of the honey can live for as long as ten thousand years." Daoist priests in this area all wished to go up there, but they all failed. The honey can only be reached by attaching a bowl-like container to the top of a bamboo pole. Yet no one was ever able to do it. Given that such inscription had been there for a long time, someone must have already visited the cave.

From *Extensive Records Compiled in the Taiping Years.*

Editor's Note:

Whether what the inscription said was true or not would never be found out, as no one was able to visit the cave and obtain the honey thereafter. It seems that such magical formula for immortality are unattainable even if they do exist.

【馬溺消腹瘕】

【原文】

昔有一人，與奴同時得腹瘕①病。奴既死，令剖腹視之，得一白鱉。乃試之諸藥澆灌之，並内②藥於腹中，悉無損動。乃系之於床脚。忽有一客來看之，乘一白馬。既而馬溺③濺鱉，鱉乃惶駭，疾走避之；既系之，不得去，乃縮藏頭頸足焉。病者察之，謂其子曰："吾病可以救矣！"乃試以白馬溺灌鱉，須臾消成水焉。病者遂頓④服升餘白馬溺，病即豁然除愈。

（選自《太平廣記 · 醫類》）

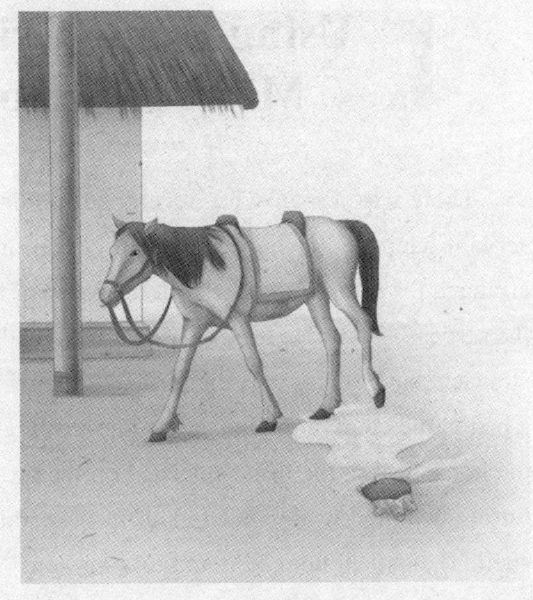

【注釋】

①腹瘕（jiǎ 假）：一種腹内疼痛結塊、散聚無常、痛無定處的疾病。至於言"剖腹視之，得一白鱉"，則是憑空想像。②内：納。③溺：同"尿"。④頓：立刻。

【釋義】

先前有一人，與他的奴僕同時患了腹瘕病。奴僕已死，便令剖腹診視，結果得一白鱉。于是嘗試着用各種藥水澆灌它，並把藥物放入它腹中，均無一點損傷。就把它拴在屋裏的床腿上。忽然有一客人乘白馬來訪，隨後馬尿濺在鱉身上，鱉於是驚駭，急忙逃走躲避；既然用繩子拴着，鱉不能離去，就把頭脚縮起來。病人觀察到這種情況，對他的兒子説："我的病可以得救啦！"於是嘗試用白馬尿灌鱉，一會兒鱉化成了水。病人就立即服一升多白馬尿，病就豁然而愈。

【按語】

本文生動地記述了用馬溺治腹瘕病的故事。雖説有些荒誕不經，但是馬溺破腹瘕，在古書上確有記載，顯然是古代的一種驗方。《本草綱目·獸部》“馬”字條云 :“白馬溺，氣味辛，微寒，有毒。主治消渴，破癥堅積聚，男子伏梁積疝，婦人瘕積。銅器承飲之。”並且還專門引用了《太平廣記》這段文字。

Using Horse Urine to Treat the Moving Tumor in the Belly

There was a man who developed moving tumors or stones in his belly, when his servant happened to have the same conditions. Following the death of the servant, he arranged for autopsy to check out the cause of the disease, only to find a white turtle inside the servant's body. He tried to use various medicines to kill it, and even put medicine in its stomach, but nothing hurt the turtle. Not knowing what to do, he had to chain the turtle to a bed in the courtyard. One day, a guest riding a white horse came to visit the man. When the horse pissed, the urine splashed on the turtle which was chained nearby. Terrified, the turtle attempted to flee but failed. In desperation, it withdrew its head and feet into the shell. The patient noticed it and told his son, "I found the cure!" He then forced the turtle to drink the urine of the white horse. A while later, the turtle melt into some kind of liquid. He then drank a sheng of horse urine and soon fully recovered.

From *Extensive Records Compiled in the Taiping Years*.

Editor's Note:

In this excerpt, the part about the white horse is quite absurd, but it was recorded in TCM texts that horse urine was effective in treating tumor or stones in the abdomen.

【應聲蟲】

【原文】

《文昌雜録》[①]：劉伯時嘗見淮西士人楊勔[②]，自言中年得異疾：每發言應答，腹中輒有蟲聲效之。數年間，其聲浸大[③]。有道士見而驚曰："此應聲蟲也，久不治，延及妻、子。宜讀《本草》[④]，過[⑤]蟲所不應者，當取服之。"勔如言，讀至雷丸[⑥]，蟲忽無聲，乃頓餌[⑦]數粒，遂愈。始未以爲信[⑧]。其後，至長汀[⑨]，遇一丐者，亦是疾，而觀者甚衆。因教之，使服雷丸。丐者謝曰："某貧，無他技，所求衣食於人者，惟藉此耳。"

應聲蟲，本病也，而丐者以爲衣食之資，死而不悔。又安知世間功名富貴，達人[⑩]不以爲應聲乎？噫，衣食誤人，肯服雷丸者鮮矣！

（選自明 · 馮夢龍《古今譚概 · 妖異部第三十四》）

【注釋】

①《文昌雜録》：書名，宋 · 龐元英撰，記録宋代元豐年間的典章制度及各種見聞。但現存《文昌雜録》無《應聲蟲》這則故事，疑是《遁齋閑覽》之誤。②劉伯時：宋人。范正敏在《遁齋閑覽》中記録這則故事時，"劉伯時"三字前有"余友"二字。楊勔（miǎn免）：宋人，不詳。 ③浸大：漸漸大起來。 ④《本草》：此指《神農本草經》。 ⑤過：當是"遇"之誤。 ⑥雷丸：中藥名，亦稱"雷矢""竹苓"。是一種寄生在竹根上的菌類。常用來驅殺人畜體内的蛔蟲等寄生蟲。 ⑦頓餌：馬上吞服。 ⑧信：真。 ⑨長汀（tīng 聽）：即今福建省長汀縣。 ⑩達人：通達的人。

【釋義】

龐元英的朋友劉伯時曾見到淮西一位讀書人楊勔，自言中年時得了一種怪病：每次一開口説話，肚子裏便跟着發出聲音，腹中有蟲應聲重復他的話。數年時間，這種聲音漸漸大起來。有位道士看到後吃驚地説："這是因爲腹中有應聲蟲的緣故，若長期不治，將會傳染給老婆孩子。我給你出個方子，你可以將《本草經》中的藥名，逐個高聲朗讀，遇到應聲蟲不敢跟着重復説出的藥名，就是醫治此蟲的良藥，當取來服用。"楊勔如法照辦，當讀到"雷丸"時，應聲蟲忽然無聲，他趕快買了雷丸服用數粒，于是病就好了。開始他不敢相信這是真的，之後，到了長汀縣，遇到了一個乞丐，也患了這種病，當時圍觀的人很多。于是便教他服用雷丸。而乞丐却謝絶説:“我貧窮,也没有别的技藝,爲了向人尋求衣食,只有依靠這個來賺錢。”

應聲蟲,本來是病呀,可是乞丐以此作爲求衣食的資本,至死而不悔。又怎麼知道,當今世間那些所謂通達之人不是把功名富貴作爲腹中的應聲蟲呢?噫!明知追求衣食富貴誤人生命,可是肯服雷丸的人少呀!

【按語】

《古今譚概》簡稱《譚概》,又名《古今笑》《古今笑史》《笑史》。筆記。明末著名文學家馮夢龍編。共三十六卷。

《應聲蟲》這則故事,由來已久,最早見於唐代張鷟的《朝野僉載》和劉餗(sù速)的《隋唐嘉話》,其後宋代范正敏所著《遁齋閑覽·人事》也有類似記載。到了明代,馮夢龍又收進《古今譚概》,並在故事的後面附上一段議論文字。顯然是用這則故事,譏諷那些不顧廉耻,不惜損害身體,而一心沉湎於功名富貴的利禄之徒。今天,我們在譏笑那些胸無主見、隨聲附和之人時,常説他是個應聲蟲。其實,應聲蟲病是可治的,可惜“肯服雷丸者鮮矣”!

雷丸,爲寄生於竹根之下的真菌菌核。它經常出現於雷雨之後,故古人認爲此物爲雷震所化,是雷神用以發霹靂的工具,且其形如彈丸,因稱雷丸。雷丸,始載於《神農本草經》,又名“雷矢”“雷實”。雷丸爲殺蟲之品,清代陳土鐸謂:“名曰雷丸者,言如雷之迅,如丸之轉也。走而不留,堅者能攻,積者能去,實至神之品。”故傳説用雷丸治愈人腹内應聲蟲。

Yesman – a Bug in the Belly

According to the Wenchang Miscellaneous Stories written by Pang Yuanying, his friend Liu Boshi once met Yang Mian, a scholar in Huaixi, who suffered a rare disease in his middle age. Every time when he said something, a bug in his belly would repeat. Year after year, the echo grew louder and louder.

A Daoist priest was startled by this, saying, "It was all because of the yesman insect in your belly. If left untreated, the disease will be passed onto your wife and children. I will tell you how to solve the problem. Read aloud the names of herbs from *King Shen Nong's Classics of Herbal Medicine*. When you encounter an herb the name of which the bug dares not repeat, you know you have found the cure." Yang did as he was told, and found that "Stone-like omphalia" was the herb that made him recover. Later, he encountered a beggar who was surrounded by a large crowd in Changting County. It turned out that the beggar also had a yesman bug in his belly. Out of sympathy for him, Yang told him about the cure. However, the beggar refused to take the medicine, saying that he was penniless and good for nothing, and marketing his weird disease was the only way for him to make a living."

The yesman bug, a rare disease that could cause one to die, was seen as an asset by the beggar. In a way, are status and wealth not the yesman in the belly of those who are wealthy and powerful? People pursue and keep such things even thought they are harmful for one's health and wellbeing. Those who are willing to take the medicine are scarce.

From *Brief Notes on the Past and Present*[1].

Notes:

1. *Brief Notes on the Past and Present* (《古今譚概》 Gujin Tangai): A collection of short stories compiled by the Ming Dynasty (1368–1644) scholar Feng Menglong.

Editor's Note:

This excerpt means to satirize people who indulge in fame and fortune at the expense of health. Today, we often mock at those who echoes and follows along whatever others say as yes-men. Actually, this disease is treatable, but people who are willing to take the medicine are scarce because everybody likes to be confirmed and agreed with.

【口吞金蠶】

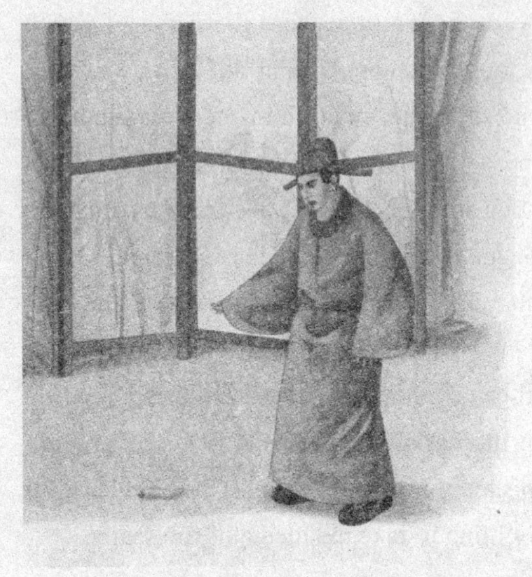

【原文】

池州[①]進士鄒閬家貧，一日啓户[②]，獲一小籠，内有銀器，持歸。覺股上有物，蠕蠕如蠶，金色燦爛，遂撥去之，仍復在舊處，踐之[③]，斫之[④]，投之水火，皆即如故。閬以問友人，友人曰："此金蠶也"。備告其故。閬歸告妻云："吾事[⑤]之不可，送之家貧，何以生爲[⑥]？"遂吞之。家人謂其必死。寂[⑦]無所苦，竟以壽終。豈至誠之盛，妖不勝正耶？

時珍竊謂金蠶之蠱，爲害甚大，故備書二事，一見此蠱畏猥，一見至誠勝邪也。

（選自明 · 李時珍《本草綱目 · 蟲部》）第四十二卷引《幕府燕閑録》）

【注釋】

①池州：地名，即今安徽省池州市。②啓户：開門。户，單扇門曰"户"。③踐之：用脚踏它。 ④斫之：用斧頭砍擊它。斫（zhúo 卓），砍，削。 ⑤事：供養，奉養。⑥何以生爲：即"以何爲生"，意爲靠什麼活着呢？ ⑦寂：很安静，平静。

【釋義】

池州進士鄒閬家境貧寒。有一天打開房門，便撿得一個小籠子，籠内裝有銀器，他就把這籠子拿回家了。這時他發現大腿上有一個東西，像蠶那樣蠕動，有金色的光澤，他把它撥在地上，但它仍回到原處。無論用脚踏、斧砍或投在水火之中，都不能把它除掉。鄒閬爲此去請教朋友，朋友説："這蟲名叫金蠶。"又詳細地告訴他關於金蠶的情況。鄒閬回家告訴他妻子説："我們養着這玩意兒不行，將帶來災難；若把金蠶送走，需很多錢財，我們家將一貧如洗，以後靠什麼生活？"于是就把那金蠶吞掉了。家人都以爲他必定會死去，但他却平平静静，没有什麼痛苦，竟然得以壽終正寢而老死家中。

難道是至誠之氣盛，自能戰勝邪妖嗎？時珍私下以爲金蠶這樣的害蟲，爲害非常嚴重，所以詳細地記録這兩件事，一是説明這種害蟲害怕刺猬，一是説明真誠可以戰勝邪妖。

【按語】

本文記述金蠶雖毒甚却不能爲害鄉閭，説明至誠之氣能够戰勝邪妖，揭示了“精誠所至，金石爲開”的道理。李時珍收載兩則金蠶的寓言故事，意在教育人心要抑惡揚善。

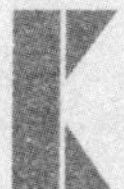

Swallowing the Golden Silkworm

Zou Lang, an advanced scholar (or Jinshi, a degree in the civil service examination system) in Chizhou, had trouble in making ends meet. One day, he found a little cage at his door. Seeing a silver container inside, he carried it home. Then he noticed that a worm-like thing with tints of gold was wriggling on his lap. He gave the worm a poke to make it fall on the ground, but it went back to his lap. He discovered that it was extremely difficult to get rid of it, for water, fire, ax or anything else can do it no harm. In desperation, he turned to his friend for help, who told him that this was the so-called Jincan, or golden silkworm. Zou went home and told his wife, “We can’t have the worm around since it will bring us disasters. However, it would cost us a large fortune to send it away and we will be left more destitute. If that’s the case, how can we survive?” He then swallowed the worm. His family thought he would soon be dead, but he was safe and sound, and died a natural death at an old age.

Was it his sincerity and integrity that made him invincible by the evil? The author believes that Jincan is truly dreadful, and that is why this story is recorded in such great details. I want to add that this worm is afraid of hedgehogs. In addition, I think sincerity can protect one from evil spirits.

From *Compendium of Materia Medica*.

Editor’s Note:

The golden silkworm is said to be highly toxic, but in this excerpt it could not harm Zou Lang. Li Shizhen recorded two fables about golden silkworm in his book to educate people to how to avoid and overcome evil forces and remain health and integrity.

【金蠶害人】

【原文】

金蠶始於蜀中，近及湖廣，閩、粵浸多[①]。狀如蠶，金色，日食蜀錦[②]四寸，南人畜之[③]，取其糞置飲食中以毒人，人即死也。蠶得所欲[④]，日置他財[⑤]使人暴富。然遣之[⑥]極難，水火兵刃所不能害。必倍其所致[⑦]，金銀錦物，置蠶於中，投之路旁，人偶收之，蠶隨以往，謂之嫁金蠶。不然能入人腹，殘齧[⑧]腸胃，完然而出，如屍蟲也。有人守福清，民訟[⑨]金蠶毒，治求不得[⑩]。或令取兩刺猬，入其家捕之必獲，猬果於榻下牆隙中擒出。夫金蠶甚毒，若有鬼神，而猬能制之何耶？

（選自明 · 李時珍《本草綱目 · 蟲部》第四十二卷引（《蔡緣叢談》））

【注釋】

①浸多：逐漸多。②蜀錦：四川産的有花紋的絲織品。③畜之：畜養它。④所欲：所需要的條件。⑤日置他財：意爲每天都能爲其主人帶來許多他人的財物。⑥遣之：送走它。⑦所致：所得到的。⑧殘齧：殘酷地咬食。齧，咬，侵蝕。⑨民訟：老百姓訴訟。⑩治求不得：想懲治他却找不到（金蠶）。治，懲處。

【釋義】

金蠶，起初在四川飼養，逐漸傳到臨近的湖北、湖南和廣西等地，後來，福建、廣東也漸漸多起來。它形狀像蠶，全身金黄色，每天需吃掉蜀錦四方寸。南方人畜養它，取它的糞便放到飲食中用來毒害人，人吃後馬上就會死去。金蠶若能得到它所需要的條件，每天都能爲主人帶來許多他人的財物，使主人突然富足。然而，送走它却很困難，即使用水淹、火燒或兵刃砍擊，也都不能絲毫損害它，一定要用倍於所得到的金銀和彩色絲織品，把金蠶放進去，拋棄在路旁，有人偶然收取這些東西，金蠶就隨着而去。這種送金蠶的辦法，叫作“嫁金蠶”。不然，金蠶能够進入人的腹内，殘酷地咬食人的腸胃，然後完整地出來，像屍蟲一樣。有一個人，叫守福清，老百姓告他用金蠶毒害人，官府要懲辦他，但在他的屋内找不到金蠶。有人獻計，讓取兩個刺猬，放入他家中一定能够捕獲金蠶，刺猬果然在床下的牆隙中將金蠶擒了出來。金蠶是極毒的東西，好像鬼神一樣，但刺猬能够制服它，這是什麼原因呢？

【按語】

本則寓言介紹了金蠶的害人習性，並說明金蠶雖毒，自然界自有相克之物，如刺猬即能制服它。

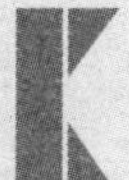 The Harmful Golden Silkworm 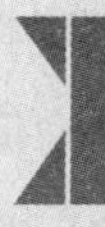

Jincan, or golden silkworm, which was first raised in Sichuan Province, and then gradually spread to neighboring Provinces of Hubei, Hunan and Guangxi. Later on, it could be found in Fujian and Guangdong. Silkworm-shaped and golden-colored, it is fed with 6 square inches of fine silk from Sichuan. Its excrement, if put in food or drink, is a deadly poison. It brings its owner considerable possessions of others, making the owner filthy rich.

It is extremely difficult to get rid of it, for water, fire, or any type of weapon can do it no harm. If the owner wants to abandon the worm, he has to put some gold or silver in a basket with the worm inside, and throw the basket away in a corner of the street, hoping someone pick it up and take it with him. This process is called "to marry off Jincan" . Otherwise, Jincan would enter the human belly, chew the stomach and intestines and then get out, just like what the so-called "corpse insect" would do.

There was a man named Shou Fuqing, who was sued by the local people for hurting others with Jincan. Due to lack of evidence, as the worm could not be found in the man's house, the government was unable to indict him. Someone suggested sending two hedgehogs to his house to catch Jincan. The worm was found as expected from the crevice in the wall below the bed. As deadly as ghosts, Jincan is curiously subdued by hedgehogs. This phenomenon is truly difficult to explain.

From *Compendium of Materia Medica*.

Editor's Note:

This excerpt describes the harmful nature and functions of golden silkworm. It is poisonous and almost impossible to subdue. Hedgehogs, however, are capable of finding and eliminating them.

【永公夢方】

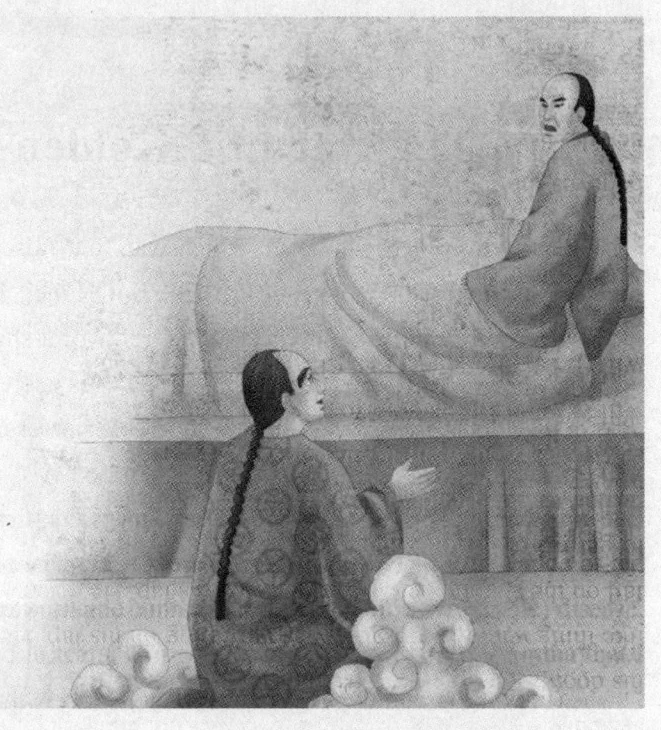

【原文】

內閣學士永公，諱①寧。嬰②疾，頗委頓③。延醫診視，未遽愈。改延一醫，索前醫所用藥帖，弗得。公以爲小婢誤置他處，責使搜索，云不得且④笞汝。方倚枕憩息，恍惚有人跪燈下曰："公勿笞婢，此藥帖小人所藏。小人即公爲臬司⑤時平反得生之囚也。"問："藏藥帖何意？"曰："醫家同類皆相忌，務改前醫之方，以見所長。公所服藥不誤，特⑥初試一劑，力尚未至耳。使⑦後醫見方，必相反以立異，則公殆矣。所以小人陰竊之。"公方昏悶，亦未思及其爲鬼。稍頃始悟，悚然⑧汗下。乃稱前方已失，不復記憶，請後醫別疏方⑨。視所用藥，則仍前醫方也。因連進數劑，病霍然如失。公鎮烏魯木齊日，親爲余言之。曰："此鬼可謂諳悉世情矣。"

（選自清・紀曉嵐《閱微草堂筆記・卷一・灤陽消夏録二》）

【注釋】

①諱：名諱。 ②嬰：遭受；纏染。 ③委頓：萎靡不振的樣子。 ④且：將。 ⑤臬司：明、清稱按察使爲臬司。 ⑥特：只。 ⑦使：假使。 ⑧悚然：恐懼的樣子。 ⑨別疏方：另開藥方。疏，開拓。

【釋義】

內閣學士永甯因病纏身，精神萎靡不振。請大夫診治，也治不好。又請一醫，此醫生索要前一醫生所用的藥方，沒有找到。永公以爲小婢放錯了地方，叫她仔細找找，並威脅說如找不到就要受鞭打。永寧靠着枕頭休息，昏睡中有個人跪在燈下，說："您不要打她，藥方是小人藏起來的，小人就是您任按察使時被您平反救活的囚犯。"永公問："你爲何藏藥方？"回答說："醫家同行相妒，他一定改前一個醫生的藥方，以顯示自己的高明。您服的藥没錯，只是剛服一劑，藥力還没發揮出來，若叫後一醫生見了藥方，他一定改前一個醫生的藥方，用相反的藥，以標新立異，那您就危險了。所以，小人偷了藥方。"永公昏昏沉沉也没想到對方是鬼。過了一會兒才猛醒過來，驚出一身冷汗。於是他說前一醫生的藥方已經丢失，找不到了，請後一醫生另開藥方。看這個醫生所用的藥，與前者一樣。於是，連服了幾劑，病很快好了。永公鎮守烏魯木齊時，親自給我講了這事，說："這個鬼真的精通人情世故啊。"

【按語】

清代紀昀所著的《閱微草堂筆記》爲筆記小说集。二十四卷。主要記述花妖狐精、鬼怪神異故事，間雜考辨，對宋儒之苛察，有所諷刺。

本文是一則寓言。不管這位永公所夢之事是真是假，但他總是得到了及時而正確的治療。這則寓言，對醫者和病者都是一個警示。

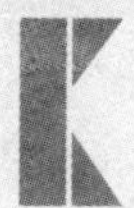

Prescription Obtained in Dream

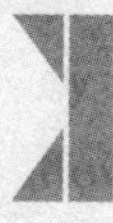

Yong Ning, an official serving in the imperial cabinet, once fell sick and was in low spirit all day long. Unsure of the doctor's capability, he sent for another. The second doctor requested for the prescription by the previous doctor, which Yong Ning had been taking medicines accordingly. It was, however, nowhere to be found. Yong blamed it on the maid, and threatened to whip her if she could not find it.As he was resting in bed leaning against pillows, he saw a man kneeling down to him next to the lamp, saying, "Please don't beat the maid, because I'm the one who hid the prescription. I was a prisoner you had saved from injustice when you were a provincial governor." Yong was surprised and asked about his motivations. The man explained, "People from the same profession always compete with one another and can never agree. Surely, the new doctor would change the prescription to appear superior. The prescription is quite all right in fact, and if you keep taking it, the medicine would prove its effectiveness. If it were to be presented to the new doctor, he will definitely revise it by prescribing medicines with opposite properties. That, however, would put your life in danger. I have no other choice but to hide it from you." Yong was daydreaming then, and he did not realize that the man was a ghost until a while later. He then felt a chill on his back. He lied to the second doctor and asked him to compose another prescription, which turned out the same as the previous one. After taking the medicine for a few days longer, Yong Ning recovered completely. When Yong Ning was later the governor of Xinjiang, he told me this story, commenting, "That ghost was sophisticated in seeing through the nature of people and human relations."

From *Writings from the Yuewei Cottage*.

Editor's Note:

This excerpt is from the book *Writings from the Yuewei Cottage* (《閱微草堂筆記》Yuewei Caotang Biji) by Ji Xiaolan (紀曉嵐 1724–1805), a famous scholar in the Qing Dynasty. Regardless of having had the dream or not, Yong Ning received timely and effective treatment. The revelation of human nature as seen from the medical profession is chilling.

參考書目
Works Cited

- Baopuzi (《抱朴子》The *Master Who Embraces Simplicity*)
- Baopuzi Neipian (《抱朴子内篇》*The Intrinsic Aspects of Embracing Simplicity*)
- Beiji Qianjin Yaofang (《備急千金要方》*Golden Prescriptions for Emergency Use*)
- Beimeng Suoyan (《北夢瑣言》*Interesting Personalities and Anecdotes from the Tang Dynasty*)
- Bencao Gangmu (《本草綱目》*Compendium of Materia Medica*)
- Bencao Shiyi (《本草拾遺》*A Supplement to the Classic of Herbal Medicine*)
- Chuyuelou Wenjianlu (《初月樓聞見録》*What I have Seen and Heard*)
- Dongjing Fu (《東京賦 》*Rhapsody of the Eastern Capital*)
- Erjing Fu (《二京賦》*Rhapsody of Eastern and Western Capital*)
- Furen Daquan Liangfang (《婦人大全良方》*Compendium of Effective Prescriptions for Women*)
- Fuzhai Riji (《復齋日記》*Diaries of Fuzhai*)
- Gengsi Bian (《庚巳編》 *A Collection of Curious Stories*)
- Guangyang Zaji (《廣陽雜記》*Miscellaneous Essays and Notes by Liu Xianting*)
- Guitian Fu (《歸田賦》*On Returning to the Fields*)
- Gujin Tangai (《古今譚概》 *Brief Notes on the Past and Present*)
- Gujin Yizhe An (《古今醫者按》*Medical Cases Past and Present*)
- Gujin Zhu (《古今注》 *Notes on Individuals and Incidents Past and Present*)
- Heguanzi (《鶡冠子》 *Heguanzi*)
- Houhanshu (《後漢書》*The Book of the Later Han*)
- Huangdi Neijing (《黄帝内經》*The Yellow Emperor's Canon of Medicine*)
- Jiayou Bencao (《嘉祐本草》*Material Medica Compled during the Jiayou Reign*)
- Jishen Lu (《稽神録》 *Deities, Spirits and Immortals*)
- Jin Shi (《金史》*History of the Jin Dynasty*)
- Jin Shu (《晉書》*The Book of the Jin Dynasty*)
- Jingzhou Ji (《荆州記》 *Records of Jingzhou*)
- Jiulingshanfang Ji (《九靈山房集》*A Collection of Works by Dai Liang*)
- Kaibao Bencao (《開寶本草》 *Materia Medica Compled during the Kaibao Reign*)

- Lenglu Yihua (《冷廬醫話》*Medical Cases Recorded in Lenglu*)
- Lingyuan Fang (《靈苑方》*Magical Formulas*)
- Liezi (《列子》*Liezi*)
- Liexian Zhuan (《列仙傳》*Biographies of Immortals*)
- Lüshi Chunqiu (《吕氏春秋》*Master Lü's Spring and Autumn Annals*)
- Mengxi Bitan (《夢溪筆談》*The Collection of Essays by Shen Kuo*)
- Mingyi Lu (《名醫録》*Biographies of Famous Doctors*)
- Muzhai Yishi (《牧齋遺事》*Past Incidents Recorded by Qian Muzhai*)
- Nandu Fu (《南都賦》*Rhapsody Southern Capital*)
- Pengchuang Leiji (《蓬窗類記》*Assorted Notes by Huang Wei*)
- Qimin Yaoshu (《齊民要術》*Essencials of People's Welfare*)
- Qianjin Fang (《千金方》*Golden Prescriptions*)
- Rihua Zi（《日華子》*Materia Medica Compiled by Rihua Zi*）
- Rumen Shiqin (《儒門事親》*Instructions on Fulfiling Fillial Piety*)
- Sandu Fu (《三都賦》*Rhapsody Three Capitals*)
- Sanguozhi (《三國志》*History of the Three Kingdoms*)
- Sanguo Yanyi（《三國演義》*Romance of the Three Kingdoms*)
- Sixuan Fu（《思玄賦》*A Contemplat Upon Mysteries*)
- Soushenji（《搜神記》*Anecdotes about Spirits and Immortals*)
- Suiyuan Shihua（《隨園詩話》*Yuan Mei's Comments of Poetry*)
- Shanghan Lun（《傷寒論》*Treatise on Febrile Diseases*)
- Shennong Bencao Jing（《神農本草經》*King Shen Nong's Classics of Herbal Medicine*)
- Shenxian Zhuan（《神仙傳》*Biographies of Divine Immortals*)
- Shiji（《史記》*Records of the Grand Historian*)
- Shishuo Xinyu（《世説新語》*A New Account of Tales of the World*)
- Shixiao Lu（《識小録》*Records of Trivial Affairs*)
- Shu Bencao（《蜀本草》*Materia Medica of the Shu Dynasty*)
- Shudu Fu（《蜀都賦》*Rhapsody of the Shu Capital*)
- Taiping Guangji（《太平廣記》*Extensive Records Compiled in the Taiping Years*)
- Taisu Mai（《太素脈》*The Taisu Pulse*)
- Tanbin Lu（《譚賓録》*A Collection of Anecdotes from the Tang Dynasty*)

- Tong Zhi (《通志》*A Comprehensive Collection of Notes and Records*)
- Bencao Tujing (《本草圖經》*Illustrated Pharmacopoeia*)
- Waitai Miyao (《外台秘要》*Arcane Essentials from the Imperial Library*)
- Wenchang Zalu (《文昌雜録》*Miscellaneous Notes Compiled by Wenchang*)
- Xijing Fu (《西京賦》*Rhapsody of the Western Capital*)
- Xiao Jing (《孝經》*Classic of Filial Piety*)
- Xinxiu Bencao (《新修本草》*Newly Revised Canon of Masteria Medica*)
- Xumoke Huixi (《續墨客揮犀》*A Sequal to Collected Notes and Essays by Peng Cheng*)
- Xunzhizhai Ji (《遜志齋集》*A Collection of Essays and Notes by Fang Xiaoru*)
- Yijianzhi (《夷堅志》*A Collection of Hearsay and Anecdotes*)
- Yijing (《易經》*The Book of Change*)
- Yi Lin (《異林》*Records of Extraordinary Things*)
- Yi Shi (《醫史》*A History of Chinese Medicine*)
- Yi Shuo (《醫説》*On Medicine*)
- Yi Yuan (《異苑》*Records of the Unusual and Curious*)
- Youyang Zazu (《酉陽雜俎》*Miscellaneous Records by Duan Chengshi*)
- Youyuzhai Yihua (《友漁齋醫話》*Huang Kaijun on Traditional Medicine*)
- Yuewei Caotang Biji (《閱微草堂筆記》*Writings from the Yuewei Cottage*)
- Zanyunlou Zashuo (《簪雲樓雜説》*Miscellaneous Essays Written on Zanyun House*)
- Zuozhuan (《左傳》*Zuo Qiuming's Commentary on Spring and Autumn Annals*)
- Zhanguo Ce (《戰國策》*Strategies of the Warring States*)
- Zhenjiu Jiayi Jing (《針灸甲乙經》*Canon of Acupuncture and Moxibustion*)
- Zhushi Jiyan Fang (《朱氏集驗方》*Effective Formulas by Doctor Zhu*)